STEPHEN CAMPOLO
PETER TZEMIS

THE 77 LAWS OF SIX PACK ABS

Disclaimer

Legal Disclaimer

Warning: All information presented in The 77 Laws Of Six Pack Abs is for educational and resource purposes only. It is not a substitute for, or addition to, any advice given to you by your physician or health care provider.

Consult your physician before making any changes to your lifestyle, diet, or exercise habits. You are solely responsible for how the information in The 77 Laws Of Six Pack Abs is perceived and utilized, and doing so is at your own risk. In no way will Peter Tzemis, Stephen Campolo, Peter Tzemis Publishing, or any persons associated with The 77 Laws Of Six Pack Abs be held responsible for any injuries or problems that may occur due to the use of this book or the advice within it.

Personal Disclaimer

I am not a doctor, and so my advice should not replace that of a doctor's. Any advice given in the book, if you choose to follow it, should be discussed between you and your doctor.

Results Disclaimer

Required Legal Disclaimer: Due to recent laws from the FTC, all companies must identify what a "typical" result is. The flat-out truth is that a typical result is nothing. No fat loss, no six pack, and no health improvements. This is because a typical person doesn't take action. The testimonials I share on various pages on my websites are not typical; they're pictures of action-takers who exercised and ate well. If you want those same results, work hard, and implement what we cover in this book.

Copyright Notice

CONTENTS

Part 2: Nutrition Laws | 45

Part 3: Training Laws | 91

To Our Former Fat-Kid Selves…
Food is good. Abs are better.

NYT BESTSELLING AUTHOR OF ENGINEERING THE ALPHA 2.0

I first met Peter in June of 2014, in a hallway outside of a conference room in Las Vegas. He was an attendee at the marketing seminar at which I'd been a speaker, and he introduced himself with a firm handshake and a gift—a book he thought I might enjoy.

Looking back now, I have no memory of what the book was, and I suspect I never got around to reading it. Still, the gesture stuck out, establishing in my mind what I would eventually come to recognize as a hallmark of Peter's personality: his willingness to go one step further, in every regard, than most people. We made our way to the lobby bar and then—four bourbons later—to the local steakhouse, where we shared our first meal together.

That dinner led to others, and eventually we ban working together, with me as his coach. This was years before he'd built name recognition as an entrepreneur. In those early days of his career, I was lucky enough to mentor him as his star was becoming ascendant in the fitness industry. Just as he had in that Las Vegas seminar, he stood out among the many people I've had the good fortune to teach over the years.

Right from the beginning, he was eager to learn, obsessed with results, and took an inquisitive eye to everything in the fitness industry at the time and asked, "why is this not working?"

Six years later, when we'd shifted from colleagues to friends and eventually to business partners, I found myself again sharing a steak (and a few bourbons) with Peter after a different seminar.

I was visiting Toronto, where I'd taught a Storytelling workshop for entrepreneurs, the attendees of which included both Peter and Stephen—who, together, co-authored the very book you now hold in your hands.

As the sun set that night, we didn't know it would be the last celebration for some time, nor the degree to which the world was about to change.

We were just entering the first stages of what Covid would unleash on the world, and in our moment of blissful ignorance, talked of lighter things. As we feasted, Peter and Stephen told me about their upcoming project: The 77 Laws of Six Pack Abs.

The book, they explained, would shed light on everything you need to get six-pack abs.

Abs, you say?

We toasted, to a new era in the fitness industry, to focus on results above jargon, to helping others first.

This is the most fulfilling part of what I do. It's getting the opportunity to work with and mentor the up-and-coming leaders of our world, support them in pushing the boundaries of their thinking, and subsequently push the industry's boundaries.

Little did we know it would be the last time we would toast in that fashion for many months.

In this book, you don't have just another fat loss book that goes on (and on) about hormones and the Krebs cycle and so forth.

That stuff's important, of course. But what separates this work from the other fat loss diet books I've seen over the last fifteen years is actionability. Peter and Stephen understand that it's not just about the information. It's about putting systems in place to actually follow the simple rules.

As the maxim goes, "Success lies in the ruthless execution of the basics."

Peter and Stephen guide through everything you could possibly need to know about how to get shredded, including the physiological details.

As a teacher, I tell writers and entrepreneurs that you have to "enter the conversation through the other person's door." You can't provide usable, practical support without understanding where your audience is coming from. Peter and Stephen understand that and craft laws to help people get shredded (and healthier). Inventive laws like "Start buying smaller clothes" line up with the tried-and-true pillars of fat loss like, get hydrated (because if you're not drinking goddam water almost, nothing else matters).

Wherever you're at in your fat loss and fitness journey, Peter and Stephen have laws for whatever door you're entering from. Start wherever strikes you, and view this as a "choose your own adventure." From the complete beginner to the seasoned meathead, there are 77 doors to open, behind which lay 77 different paths to choose. From there, you can build off the ones that first strike you and continue to integrate more and more laws into your life.

Finally, I admire how these two keep in mind that fat loss isn't everything, or even the end goal: it's the means to a better, happier, healthier life. They tackle issues like depression in ways most diet books never touch.

Writing this—nearly a year later—, the world is a different place than when we feasted in Toronto. Covid has upended so much of our culture, revealed our weaknesses, and brought us to our knees in many respects.

It's also shown us how much of what we want (and have always wanted) is to feel in control of ourselves and our health.

As I read through some of these laws, I was reminded of a lesson I learned through a lifetime of mental health struggles and decades in fitness: a six-pack won't make your problems go away—you still have to deal with them. In the face of a global pandemic, sometimes "vanity" seems silly.

But finding ways to improve yourself so you can improve the world, finding reasons to be healthy—well, there's no downside.

Because even when it seems the world is ending, having a six-pack feels cool. And that's reason enough.

-JR

PART 1

MINDSET LAWS

"You cannot solve your problems with the same mindset you used to create them."

—*ALBERT EINSTEIN*

BEFORE YOU CAN even think of building a house, you need to lay a solid foundation. And, likely one with reinforced concrete and steel to handle the strain and new changes to the land, all while ensuring the stability and safety of the constructor for eternity. It's no surprise, then, that contractors spend up to 80% of the time building a foundation, before adding everything else.

Six pack abs are no different. And our foundation begins in the mind. Because no diet, exercise program, or fat loss pill can overcome limiting beliefs and self-sabotage. If they could, you probably wouldn't be reading this book, and Stephen and I would be out of a job.

Backed by centuries of real-life experience, these first 22 mindset laws will help conquer your inner demons and give you the six pack shortcut.

LAW #1
TAKE RESPONSIBILITY

THE BIGGEST REASON people don't reach their goals is they've played the victim their whole lives and can't accept blame. If you're fat, it's your fault. If you're broke, it's your fault. If you're alone, it's your fault. I know it's harsh, but I'm not here to pat you on the ass and tell you what you want to hear.

As a fitness coach who has worked with thousands of clients, those who achieve the biggest transformations are the ones who accept responsibility. They realize that their actions and crappy lifestyle have gotten them where they are today.

On the flip side, the clients who rarely get results are the ones who blame everything on someone else. Their girlfriend made them go out to eat. Their mom cooked their favorite meal and they couldn't resist. It was their friend's birthday, and they wanted to drink and party. The list goes on.

Nobody is responsible for your life but you. Nobody is coming to save you. If you want to play the victim and blame the world for your problems, then you will continue to get the same results.

Own your life. Own your decisions. Take responsibility. If you can do this, then you have taken the first step towards transforming. Once you accept responsibility, you will have the power to change your life and make the right decisions towards a better life.

CREATE A NEW SELF-IMAGE

MY HYPOTHESIS IS simple: at this very moment, you know exactly what you need to do to level up your life. You already know the "secrets" to have more money, better relationships, more productivity, and a shredded six pack, and yet you don't execute a plan.

For the longest time, we believed a lack of discipline and willpower were the culprits. But, that's only part of the answer. We're only governed by willpower when we actively focus on what we're doing, which is only a few times a day when we do things that aren't habitual. The rest of the time, we function on autopilot.

Our habitual behavior is controlled by our self-image. This self-image dictates our habits, and our habits determine our long-term results.

Maxwell Maltz, a famous psychologist in the 1960s, wrote a book called Psycho-Cybernetics. He spent his entire life studying the way a person's image and perception of themselves shape their results in life. He concluded that self-image controls our results, just like a cybernetic mechanism.

Take a thermostat, for example. If you set the temperature to 78 degrees, then anytime the temperature rises or falls below that number, the thermostat kicks in to bring the temperature back to

78 degrees. When you try to lose weight, more often than not, you'll unconsciously return to your set point.

There are two big ways to change your self-image:

1. A POWERFUL EMOTIONAL EVENT

We've all heard about those people that completely changed their lives after a powerful experience. A car accident, the loss of a loved one, public humiliation, an unexpected victory, having a baby, losing your home - any of these incidents can be life-changing.

But we can't control this. So, instead of waiting for something like this to happen to motivate us to change our lives, we're going to use the other way.

2. AUTOSUGGESTION: CONSTANT SPACED REPETITION OF YOUR GOAL

This is when you repeat an idea or image for so long that it becomes your normal way of thinking. Besides emotional shock, it is the only known method of influencing the subconscious mind.

The best way I have found to ensure successful autosuggestion is to carry around and read a goal card every day. This method will engrain your goal so deeply into your mind that you will unconsciously start to act towards the attainment of your goal.

Here's what your goal card should look like on the front:

Insert Goal Here and
the Date to Achieve It By

- Daily Action Step #1
- Daily Action Step #2
- Daily Action Step #3
- Daily Action Step #4

Here's what your goal card should look like on the back:

Insert Goal Here and the
Date to Achieve It By

- Description of your life when you achieve the goal. Make sure to include your feelings, daily process and how amazing life is now that you have achieved it.
- Picture of goal (if possible)

Keep it in your pocket at all times and read it every morning and night. Personally, I read mine every time I go to the bathroom as well. Over time, you'll start to notice that this piece of paper becomes your reality. Eventually, you can expand your goals to go beyond six pack abs and really watch the magic of this goal card unfold.

Another highly effective way of applying autosuggestion is by repeating self-affirmations when you get up and before you go to bed. I typically do this while staring at myself in the mirror, almost in a way where I am commanding myself with 100% certainty who I am and what I have. Even if you don't have it yet, you must believe it as if it were already in your possession.

My daily affirmations look something like this:

1. I am powerful beyond measure
2. I can accomplish anything I set my mind to
3. I accept what I cannot change
4. I have control over my thoughts, feelings, and choices
5. I am in complete control of my life
6. I am loved
7. I am disciplined
8. I am healthy and fit
9. My body craves healthy and nutritious foods
10. I do hard things because I am willing to pay the price for greatness

DEFINE SUCCESS BEFORE YOU CHASE IT

LET ME TELL you the story of the failed Gold Medalist, Corrine Archer. By the age of 7, she had already logged hundreds of hours of training in pursuit of an Olympic title. At the age of 17, after ruthlessly training for over a decade, she won her much-coveted Olympic gold medal.

By anyone's definition, Corinne Archer was a success story. What she had spent two-thirds of her life pursuing, she finally obtained. She had the gold medal to prove it. However, Corinne left the podium not in tears of joy, but with a gnawing sense of emptiness. It took several painful months before Corinne began to come to terms with the shock of losing a goal by winning it.

Success, then, is not a trophy we seize, a record we set, or a position we earn. It's not the figures in our bank account, the zipcode we live at, or the shredded six pack we can show off. True success — the kind which doesn't slip through your fingers the moment you get hold of it — is part of a continuous journey rather than an endpoint. Before even beginning this process of getting in the best shape of your life, you must realize that there is no finish line. There will always be something you want to change. This is good because it keeps you motivated and hungry.

All your efforts should be focused on achieving a successful life, whatever that looks like for you specifically. Only you know what a "successful life" really is. Too many people on their journey to six pack abs, forget to build six pack abs into their life instead of the other way around.

They quickly find out that having a six pack comes at a cost far greater than it's worth. This is why it's critical to choose specific goals that reflect the life you want to live. Map out your goals so far ahead of their deadlines that you have plenty of time to evolve into the person who deserves them. If not, success will pay you an infrequent visit, if it comes at all.

Before you spend several months or years hunting for six pack abs (or any other type of "success"), spend a few minutes defining what it really means to you.

LAW #4

RESPECT THE TIMELINE

MOST PEOPLE DON'T understand how long it will take to get visible abs. It takes most people years to get out of shape and overweight or obese, but after a few days of dieting and exercising, they expect to see instant shredded abs. Did you get fat overnight? Of course not. So don't expect to get shredded overnight either. Like all things in life, it takes time and patience.

The chart below is a pretty accurate description of how long it will take to see your abs based on where you currently are.

Starting Body Fat % Weeks Until Six Pack Abs

10-13%	4 Weeks Or Less
14-16%	8 Weeks
17-18%	12 Weeks
19-20%	16 Weeks
21-23%	24 Weeks
24-26%	32 Weeks
27-29%	40 Weeks
30%+	52 Weeks Or More

Now, the actual amount of time it's going to take can be slightly more or less depending on how well you stick to your diet and training program, whether you use supplements to speed up the process, and how efficiently or inefficiently your body tends to mobilize and burn fat.

That being said, most people underestimate how long it's really going to take to get in amazing shape. If you want to achieve it as fast as possible, then being consistent with your diet and training will get you where you want to be in the shortest amount of time.

Consistency will be your biggest asset.

LAW #5

KNOW YOUR "TRUE" BODY FAT PERCENTAGE

THERE'S A TREND that has emerged recently that needs to die. If you believe social media or the common gym talk, nobody that lifts is any higher than 12-15% body fat, regardless of how lean they look. And, never have I heard of so many people being "6-8%".

In fact, if you "are" 10%, well you're actually kind of fat

What is the problem, you may ask? Who cares if everybody lies (or is just misinformed) about their body fat levels?

1. **It can give you unrealistic expectations.** If you think that you are 12% body fat, you might "believe" that you are only 5-10lbs away from looking shredded. When you lose 10lbs and still don't look great, it might kill your motivation.

2. **It provides false programming.** Your daily caloric intakes rely on knowing your body fat percentage. By not knowing your true body fat percentage, you're setting yourself for failure.

So, how does one accurately measure their body fat percentage? Many coaches and "gurus" recommend body fat calipers. I disagree. Unless someone is a trained technician in Caliper reading, you will most likely have a faulty body fat percentage reading.

One time when I was getting ready for a shoot, I was assessed by five different professional coaches. Each time I got five different bodyfat percentages ranging from 7% - 14%.

So what should you do instead? Get a DEXA scan. They can be hard to find, but they are a game changer.

The whole process takes about 15min, and you'll have 99.5% accurate picture of what's going on inside your body.

Another, more plebeian approach, is to visually assess yourself based on pictures. In reality, nobody but you cares about what your body fat percentage is. You should only use it to create a proper nutrition and training program.

IMG

Remember, you don't need to be at 8% to be ripped. Some guys look just as shredded at 12% then they do at 8%.

But knowing your honest starting point will stop you from sabotaging your quest before you even start.

LAW #6
WRITE OUT 100 REASONS

N 1993, MICROSOFT started an online encyclopedia called Encarta. They had professionals write and edit thousands of articles with entire teams overseeing the project.

A few years later, Wikipedia appeared on the scene, but with a different model. People were invited to write articles because they wanted to and nobody was paid a cent. Ten years ago, if you had to predict which model was going to win, I'm sure you would've bet on Encarta.

Wikipedia won by a landslide, and it's all because they had the right type of motivation. Without a doubt, internal motivation beats external motivation every single time. The Wikipedia writers did it because they genuinely wanted to. Their work had a sense of purpose, and you can see it. Internal motivation is often the missing ingredient to achieving six pack status. Unfortunately, we've never really been taught how to create internal motivation for our own goals. We grow up in a society that punishes us for creativity and rewards us for conforming.

As a kid, you listened to your teachers and parents. At your job, your boss's word is law. We've been programmed to rely on authority for direction and devalue our own commands. If the president of your country came to you and said, "We require you to get lean, the country depends on you," you'd do it. But when you give yourself a command, you often slack off, like your words don't hold any value.

This is wrong. You must be able to give meaning to your goals yourself and not wait for an authority to do it for you. You must be able to create so much internal motivation that you would stay up all night working on your goals.

Here's a simple method to get you started on the right path. Grab a pen and paper and write out 100 reasons why you want to achieve your goal (six pack abs) on a piece of paper. Now go put it somewhere you can see it daily.

You may say, 'but Peter, I can't write 100 reasons, I can barely write 10.' Well, that's the problem. You don't care about your goal enough. Sit down and think really hard about why you want to be in shape. Don't give up until you get to 100.

When you're done, email them to peter@petertzemis.com

LAW #7
MEDITATE

ALMOST EVERY SUCCESSFUL person I've ever had the great fortune of meeting practices some form of meditation on a daily basis.

Meditation is essentially a mind bath. It helps cleanse all the crap that's built up in our day-to-day lives. It allows us to gain altitude over our lives, to see our lives from a 30,000-foot view. Meditation allows us to regain control. By taking one step back, meditation allows us to leap three steps forward.

The best way I have found to start meditating consistently is by using an app called Headspace. Headspace provides daily 10-minute audio recordings that guide you along a meditative process. It's free for the first ten days, but once you start, you'll quickly get addicted to the feeling.

Another option, if you can't possibly find ten minutes extra per day, is to follow the program '3-minute meditations' by my friend, Adam Michael Brewer (petertzemis.com/meditate).

It's doable, realistic, time-friendly, and all-inclusive.

Meditation will provide you with physical, mental, and emotional harmony. And thus, make six pack abs effortless.

LAW #8
RAISE YOUR STANDARDS

CONRAD HILTON, FOUNDER of Hilton hotels, once said: "I do not know anything that will halt life success faster than self-satisfaction and low standards."

A standard is a level of living that you consider to be your minimum to be happy. The standards you set always get met. No matter what. In the past, I'm willing to bet your standards for having six pack abs were: I'm going to try to get a six pack. If your standard was: I will accept nothing less than having a shredded six pack, you probably wouldn't even be reading this book.

Whatever you have in your life, or whatever you're working towards, the point at which you take your foot off the gas pedal is your standard.

Now, the problem is that you can't just set absurd standards right now. It's more of an art. If your standards are too high without sufficiently progressing towards them in a reasonable amount of time, you end up with self-loathing.

Raise them high enough, but not to a ridiculous height.

If you're 50lbs overweight, start by setting your standard to weigh 15lbs less. Once you achieve that goal, set a new standard of weighing 30lbs less. Once you achieve that, you can set a goal of getting a four-pack. Before you know it, you'll have your six pack, and your standards will be permanently set there.

Here are the four steps I use to instill a higher standard for myself and my clients.

1. Get environmental exposure. Hang around people who have shredded six packs. Observe their lives closely and how people react to them. Once you experience it up close, you'll feel either inspiration, desperation, or both.
2. Make a real decision. Failure is not an option. Get obsessed with achieving the goal you've set.
3. Set a massive goal reward. For me, it's usually a kick-ass vacation to somewhere new or a photoshoot.
4. Re-raise your standard once you hit it. Too many times, people achieve their goal and take their foot off the gas pedal. Instead, I challenge you to re-raise that standard. Did you hit your six pack goal? Great. Now keep it for six weeks while eating more food. Did you make $100k? Good, now go after 250k. Raise your standards, improve your life.

Once you stop raising the bar in your life, you will regress…and slowly but surely, you will wind up right back where you started. Never become complacent, and never, ever settle.

Settling means you're dead.

LAW #9
CREATE A COMEBACK STORY

AS I'M WRITING this, the Coronavirus pandemic is currently shutting down the world. The economy is crashing. Here in Florida, where I live, they've just issued a mandatory stay-at-home order for the next 30 days. Small business owners are going bankrupt. Employees have no income. People are losing their jobs, homes, and cars. Things are dire and depressing, to put it mildly. But here is the thing, as bad as things are, and as horrible as this current situation is for everyone around the world, it offers an opportunity for one thing: A Comeback Story.

The world is going through an awakening. People are being forced to reinvent themselves and reflect on what is actually important. Many people are using this opportunity to get healthy, get fit, and strengthen their immune system. But on the flip side, you have people sleeping in, watching Netflix and YouTube all day, and literally wasting away.

Many people will emerge from this crazy time in history with an amazing comeback story. Stories of triumph and resiliency. Sadly, many other people will come out of this time weaker, fatter, and worse off than when they went in.

You see, everyone has the opportunity to create their own comeback story, yet many people will never take advantage of it.

The reason I don't regret being 100 pounds overweight when I was younger is because it's part of my comeback story. Being fat was the foundation I needed to overcome. I can relate to overweight people. I can relate to the fat kid getting picked on because that was part of my story too. But, I overcame. And guess what? You can too.

Take a good look in the mirror. No, seriously. Put the book down, get up, and look in the mirror. Today could be the worst you ever look for the rest of your life. Each day after today, you can write your story however you want. Make a choice and decide that you deserve better. Every day is a day closer to your dream body and your dream life…if…and only if…you decide you're worth it.

LAW #10

SCHEDULE A NON-REFUNDABLE PHOTOSHOOT OR BEACH VACATION

COMMITMENT TAKES COURAGE. Many times, we are content to stand on the sidelines and simply watch the game being played. It's safer there, but there's no action and no opportunity for success or growth. Sometimes, we just need to jump into it and see what happens. Sometimes, we just need to burn the boats. The ancient Greek warriors understood this idea.

The Greeks possessed an unwavering attitude to victory and commitment. When the Grecian armies landed on their enemy's shore, the first order the commanders gave was to "burn the boats." These commanders knew the power of motivation. With no boats to retreat to, the army had no choice but to be successful to survive. As the soldiers watched the boats burn, they knew there was no turning back – there would be no surrendering.

"If you want to take the island, burn the boats."

People often don't get abs because they don't have enough motivation. They don't have anything on the line. You need to have skin in the game. Scheduling a paid upfront and non-refundable photoshoot or a beach vacation gives you a point of no return. It's the six pack version of burning your boat. Leave your fear and regret at the bottom of the water with the boat and begin moving in the direction you want to go. Surrender to no one and fully commit. You will be victorious.

START BUYING SMALLER CLOTHES

WHEN I DECIDED I wanted to get really lean and under 10% body fat, the first thing I would do is take a trip to my favorite clothing stores. But…I would buy clothes one size smaller.

If my waist size was 34, I would purposely buy a pair of jeans I love but in a size 32 waist. The same thing goes for shirts. I would find some shirts I really love and buy them in a size smaller than I usually was. If I'm currently wearing an extra-large shirt, then I would buy a large shirt.

When I got home, I would hang the clothes up somewhere I was going to see them every day. When I woke up, I would see them, when I went to bed, I would see them. This keeps me motivated to get in shape and get lean so I can wear my new jeans and new shirts.

LAW #12

JOURNAL NIGHTLY

YOU KNOW YOU want abs, but you can't seem to get there. You know the laws, but doing them is hard. Some days, it seems more realistic to just give up entirely. The whole taking one step forward and one or two steps backward pattern is getting old.

When there's a gap between who you are and who you intend to be, you are unhappy. You're torn, mentally exhausted, and regretful. You always feel a little like a fraud to yourself, and probably to the people around you.

More effective than microscopically analyzing your sabotaging behaviors, is nailing down a "keystone" habit that tightly locks all of your other habits in place. Without the keystone, everything falls apart.

Journaling nightly is that keystone.

Keystone habits spark a chain reaction of other good habits and can rapidly alter every aspect of your life.

Here's how we do six pack journaling. Answer the following questions in your journal every single night before bed (with pen and paper is better):

1. What went well today?
2. What could I improve?
3. How can I make tomorrow awesome?

If done effectively, journaling will change everything in your life for the better.

You'll become the person you want to be. You'll design the life you want to live. Your relationships will be healthier and happier. You'll be more productive and powerful. You'll unlock your six pack.

Journal nightly.

LAW #13
GET OBSESSED

MANY OF MY life philosophies contradict the normal "blue pill" underpaid 9-5, high-fructose-corn-syrup-fed, mind-numbed, creativity-void, undersexed, out-of-shape average-guy mentalities.

Many of them even directly contradict the accepted "foundations" of mainstream self-improvement, which is otherwise a significant upgrade to an "average guy" life.

This law does both.

Anything that I (or my ultra-successful clients and friends) ever accomplished in life is a product of obsession, not moderation.

Thinking about my goal when I wake up. Thinking about my goal when I make my six pack shake in the morning. Thinking about my goal when I brush my teeth. Thinking about my goal when walking to the gym. Thinking about my goal when I'm at the grocery store. Thinking about my goal when I'm putting food in the fridge. Thinking about my goal when I'm drinking a protein shake. Thinking about my ONE GOAL when I'm getting ready for bed.

You get the point.

The word "obsession" has a negative connotation and obviously, it's not a good idea to obsess over things you don't like. A lot of people somehow believe that investing nearly all your physical and psychological time and energy into ONE thing is a bad idea.

Guess why we have so many average people in the world?

Get obsessed with your six pack. Find a plan and take action. Stop reading my fucking book and go make something happen (please come back later… thank you).

LAW #14

CRUSH NEGATIVITY AND DEPRESSION

HAD A MASSIVE problem with negativity and jealousy until I was 23 years old. The ironic thing is that I didn't even know it. Negativity can take years off your life, prevent you from accomplishing your goals, and even make you fatigued and fat (cortisol). The good news is, it can be beat.

1. **Admit that you are a negative person (and it's negatively affecting your life)**

2. **Distance yourself from negative people and toxic relationships** - Every day you spend with negative people filling your thoughts is a step backward. You aren't going to change them — that has to be internal. Whether you ditch them today or tomorrow is up to you, but to live an epic life and reclaim your six pack, you will have to distance yourself.

3. **Stop being sarcastic** - Sarcasm is often a form of negativity, even if it's funny, it needs to be limited. Not always, but sarcasm tends to come from a form of deep-seated bitterness (as was the case for me). Avoid doing it as much as possible.

4. **Stop being a hater** - Haters are jealous, negative people. These days, it's much more acceptable and popular to try and tear people down rather than speak positively about them. One of the better ways to break this cycle is to be working on a worthwhile goal where you literally don't have the urge or time to be a jealous chump. If the urge to be jealous comes, instead, ask yourself what you can learn from this person to help improve your own life.

5. **Give yourself a break** - Guys like us tend to punish ourselves too hard when something goes wrong. Instead, realize that "wrong" is just a temporary condition and take responsibility by fixing it.

Negativity goes beyond just a situational mindset. It's a lifestyle and definitely not a healthy one. It can even be a symptom of low-level depression. If you have depression (or think you do), your first priority is to beat the depression.

Both these things will destroy your life, your six pack, and hinder any effort toward improving them. As a side note, I've never met a really negative person with a solid six pack.

Coincidence?

LAW #15
STOP WATCHING PORN

USED TO LOVE porn. What guy doesn't? An endless stream of hot, naked women, all just a click away. If something is too good to be true, it often is.

Research has shown that porn use can change the neural pathways of the brain, causing addiction, hormonal changes, and sexual dysfunction. Studies show between a 600% and 3000% increase in erectile dysfunction among young men since the emergence of internet pornography (I get hundreds of emails alone every year about this).

Porn use has also been shown to mess with your delicate brain chemical balance (your neurotype) as well as destroy your testosterone, ambition, and motivation - the very essence of what a man is.

More insidious than the physical effects of porn addiction is its reported effects on the addict's emotional and psychological well-being. Long-term porn users have been shown to prefer porn over sex with real people. They're also more at risk for violence, depression, obesity, and drug addiction.

If that doesn't scare you enough to quit porn today and never look back, let's look at the superpowers of rebooting - the process of recovering from pornography damage.

1. Confidence boost
2. Increased sexual interest from others
3. Creative mojo
4. Social awareness
5. Reduced anxiety and shame
6. More free time
7. Better sexual function
8. Super recovery - attributed to testosterone-enhancing benefits of nofap.
9. Extreme will power
10. Laser focus

If it isn't abundantly clear yet, you need to stop watching porn immediately. Do not seek out and watch pornographic material either as video, image or text, both online and offline. This includes services like Chatroulette or online dating websites or apps.

It's fucking awful for you and will destroy any chance you have at building a kickass six pack and an amazing life.

Plus, sex with real people is much better.

LAW #16
GET UNCOMFORTABLE BEING COMFORTABLE

U NDERACHIEVEMENT IS NOT caused by the usual suspects: lack of work ethic, lack of opportunity, or lack of talent. The reason most people don't succeed with (insert your goal here) is far more obvious and far more pathetic.

It's the reason why you'll never get your six pack, reach your dating goals, or become financially free (whatever that means).

In hindsight, it was my biggest obstacle too.

It was something I struggled with and still do to this day, although to a far lesser degree. The problem is, you live a comfortable life.

Admit it.

Your life is simply too comfortable for you to make the necessary physical and psychological changes in your life. For many men (especially the younger guys), 21st-century mediocrity isn't particularly uncomfortable. In fact, many secretly enjoy it (I know I used to).

Instinctually and logically, your mind tries to keep your life as stress and pain-free as possible. Your mind and body won't even want to go to the gym or eat healthy until you force them to.

Even if you aren't overly privileged, you probably live a comfortable life. You might argue otherwise, citing your boring social life, job, or mediocre relationships, but overall, you know your life is pretty comfortable.

There's plenty of porn, video games, and Netflix to keep you from hitting rock bottom, which would otherwise force you to be accountable for all those wasted hours. You're just comfortable enough to do what ultimately amounts to nothing and be happy with your effort.

That type of comfortable approach to life isn't going to cut it if you want to be on top (and reap the benefits of being there).

To quote one of my favorite authors, "It won't be a lack of opportunity, a lack of work ethic and won't even be a lack of talent that will kill most of your dreams (and your abs), it's the highly comfortable, mediocre life that you are accustomed to."

Acquire an authentic disdain for the comfortable majority and watch your six pack (and other goals) come to life faster than you could've ever thought.

LAW #17
KEEP BUSY

ONE OF THE big problems with getting in shape is that it's hard to eat so little, for so long. Your body hates it. The secret to making it effortless? Keep busy.

When you're busy, your mind is focused on things other than the lack of food your body is getting. Time flies by without a hint of hunger.

Before you know it, it's dinner time, and you've got a huge 1200 calorie buffer to play with.

If you aren't naturally busy, force yourself. Volunteer. Get a second job. Pet sit. Whatever it takes, get busy.

Getting into (and staying in) my best shape was easiest when I was starting my company in university. Between work, school, and enjoying university life, there was no time to pig out — nor was there really a need to.

We often cheat on our diets as a remedy for something else in our lives (as we discuss in law #61. When you become ultra-busy, your life will improve, you'll be happier, and your abs will appear.

BEAT THE WINDOW OF INTENSITY

WHETHER YOUR CRAVINGS are physiological or psychological, there's a window of time where the cravings will be at their peak and when you are most triggered. We call this:

THE WINDOW OF INTENSITY.

The window of intensity (WIN) lasts about 15 minutes, on average. That doesn't mean it will always be limited to 15 minutes, just that 15 minutes is roughly what you should expect in most scenarios. In this window, you will experience justifications, rationalizations, self-talk, and so on. Don't be caught off guard when you experience this, because on your journey to reach low levels of body fat; it'll happen daily, so you need to make sure you prepare for it.

I like the acronym "WIN" because it's easy to remember when you get triggered, and it alludes to this small window of time that you must overcome to reach your fat-loss goals. When you find yourself being triggered, "WIN" should pop into your head.

If you've already prepared your environment for success, and have removed any temptations or trigger foods, then chances are you will succeed at getting through the WIN successfully, for the simple fact that you don't have any processed, hyper-palatable foods at your disposal.

However, there's still a chance that you will seek some sort of "real" but also hyper-palatable food (peanut butter anyone?) during this time. If the craving isn't fed after about 15 minutes, it begins to rapidly decline in influence. Most people who are triggered immediately feed the craving. Your goal is to institute specific delays that are also designed to help you navigate the WIN until it stops manipulating you.

Here are three strategies I teach my clients:

1. Drinking a glass of ice cold water, a cup of tea, etc. is a great first start as it allows you to put something in your stomach (which can also fill a physiological need. If you are dehydrated you can experience WIN because your body craves water).

2. Brush your teeth. We associate brushing with finishing a meal and doing it signals to the brain that there is no more eating.

3. If possible, leave the situation. If you're in the office, go outside for five minutes. At home, I recommend jumping in the shower or washing your face (although you can take a walk too).

The main thing you need to do is change your immediate environment. I sound like a broken record, but it's important that you understand this:

Destroy temptation by eliminating any trigger foods from your environment.

If you can do this, reaching your physique goals will be so much easier.

LISTEN TO THE "HUMAN" BRAIN

HAVE YOU EVER had an internal dialogue with yourself? It's almost as if you have two different voices arguing back and forth in your head. One voice is speaking to your higher self, trying to bring out the greatness in you by getting you to do the things you don't want to do, but will make you better as a person. The other voice wants you to be lazy, eat garbage, and give into any immediate gratification.

There is a reason we all experience this. It's because we are at constant battle between our two brains:

The **animal brain** and the **human brain**.

The Animal Brain, also known as the "reptilian brain," only cares about survival. Anything related to thirst, hunger, and sexual urges. Your animal brain wants you to eat garbage food and stay chubby because this ensures your survival. The animal brain doesn't realize it's 2020, and food is everywhere. Unfortunately, this works against you when you're trying to get lean. So you start to justify why you deserve the piece of chocolate or the cookie or the brownie. Eventually, you talk yourself into it, and you end up eating the entire package and ruin your progress.

Your human brain is responsible for emotions and reasoning. For example, have you ever wanted to have that chocolate donut, but there's an internal voice that tells you not to do it because you're going to regret it? That's your human brain. This is the part of your brain you need to listen to.

Here's the cool thing...you can train yourself to silence your animal brain. Just like anything, it takes practice. You need to practice overcoming those urges and instincts to go raid your pantry and fridge at night when you have sugar cravings. The more you overcome these situations, and the more wins you have over the animal brain, the less loud that part of your brain will be.

So stop allowing your animal brain to control your life and habits. Overcome it by depriving it of what it wants. Allow the human brain to take over and dictate your choices and decisions.

LAW #20
MANAGE THE WEEKEND

YEARS AGO, MY fitness coach told me something I've never forgotten. He said, "never let the weekend be your weak end."

For a long time, I was on this crazy rollercoaster. Monday through Friday, I would bust my ass in the gym. I would be extremely strict with my diet and nutrition, and I would make progress. Then, the weekend came. I treated the weekend like a free for all. I ate what I wanted, drank what I wanted, and didn't count a single calorie. I sabotaged all of my hard work from the week before. When Monday morning would come, it was like I was starting all over again. This went on for years and years because I had no plan and no structure on the weekend.

For most people, they do great during the week with their nutrition and training. But when the weekend comes, everything falls apart. Why does this happen? Well, during the week, most of us have structure. We wake up at a certain time, we get to work at a certain time, we eat at a certain time, we workout at a certain time...we have a routine and things are planned. When the weekend comes, and this structure is no longer there, it becomes much harder to stay accountable to your diet and training because you are out of your routine. So how do we fix this? We add structure to our weekend and plan things out.

I have more structure and safeguards in place during the weekend than I do during the week, as I am a lot more likely to cheat on my diet during the weekend. Most people are off from work and there are more social events happening, so it's much easier to just give in and enjoy yourself. There is nothing wrong with enjoying yourself…but you must plan for it.

On Saturday, I always wake up early and go to the gym. If I sleep in, the odds of me actually going to the gym are slim, so this is a non-negotiable that I have. This way, my workout is out of the way.

Now, keeping nutrition on track is where people struggle most. Dinner with friends, birthday parties, drinks, appetizers, pizza and wings, beer, bottomless mimosas with Sunday brunch…the temptation is everywhere. You need to pick and choose what you enjoy.

For example, if I have dinner with friends planned on Saturday night, then I will simply fast until 4 pm that day. I will then break my fast with an apple and a protein shake, which will hold me over until dinner. For dinner, I will enjoy myself and order what I want and have a few beers. All I am doing is saving my calories for later in the day so I can enjoy myself. Planning for things is how you can have your cake and eat it too…or pizza or burritos. This is how you master the weekend.

Going into the weekend, if you fail to plan, then plan to fail.

PLAN YOUR TRAVEL

THERE ARE TWO situations where I see people go off track with their nutrition and training and destroy all their progress.

1. During the weekend
2. When they travel

What do both of these have in common? Lack of structure and planning. I sound like a broken record, but you need to understand this, if you fail to plan then you can plan to fail.

Traveling, either for pleasure or business, can be challenging for anyone. There's no structure or set schedule like there is when you're at home, so you need to hold yourself much more accountable when you travel, and you need to be intentional about every single choice you make when it comes to your nutrition.

Whenever I have an early morning flight, I will always do intermittent fasting. I have a cup of coffee or two before my flight, along with a good amount of water. This will typically keep me full until noon. If I have a layover and I'm hungry, I will have a protein bar and some more coffee. I don't like to eat big meals in airports because the food selection typically isn't the greatest, and the food at the airport is so damn expensive.

Now, if I have an afternoon or evening flight, then I will have a large meal beforehand. For example, let's say I'm flying from Florida to California and my flight is at 4 pm. The total flight time is about seven hours (including the two-hour layover), so I want to eat something that's going to fill me up and keep me full for the entire time I'm traveling. This is why my pre-travel meal of choice is always a ton of greens and a source of protein. I usually have a huge salad with about a pound of lean meat (turkey, chicken, or ground beef). The salad has practically no calories and is a high volume of food. Eating low-calorie, high-volume foods is key. Protein is very satiating, so combining protein with a lot of greens is a great combination to keep your stomach full for hours. I typically won't be hungry for 6-8 hours after eating this meal.

Now, once you finally reach your destination and get settled in, you want to try to keep your body in the same rhythm as when you are home. If you exercise in the morning, then continue to exercise in the morning. If your hotel doesn't have weights, then go for a jog or a walk. Just move your body for 30-60 minutes. Working out while on vacation is amazing for releasing endorphins and getting you in the right mental state.

The problem when people travel is they stop exercising and start eating like crazy, so they feel like garbage. You want to avoid this at all costs. If you know you're going to be eating more and drinking more on your trip, then make sure you get your exercise in during the morning to offset some of those extra calories.

Also, continue practicing intermittent fasting. Save the majority of your calories for later in the day when you go to dinner. Having coffee and drinking sparkling water throughout the morning and early afternoon will help keep your stomach full.

The same applies for when you're traveling for business. If you know you have nice dinners with clients planned, then fast that morning and have a lighter lunch to hold you over. If you plan for these, you'll succeed.

When it comes to traveling and reaching your fitness goals, if you don't have a plan, you will get back from your trip 5-10 pounds heavier, and you will need a month just to get back to where you were. Trust me; I've done this numerous times.

LAW #22
DON'T EAT IN FRONT OF THE TV

THE EASIEST WAY to overeat and pack on body fat is by being distracted when eating. Whether that's eating in front of the TV, scrolling through Instagram, or watching your favorite TV show on your computer, it needs to stop now.

Distracted eating contributes to weight gain, a sedentary lifestyle, and overall unhealthiness, not to mention an inability to reach low levels of body fat. This is mainly because distracted eating screws up your brain chemicals when you sit down to feast.

When you eat, your brain registers that nutrition is entering your body. It then starts to send chemicals to indicate a level of fullness. When we eat while distracted, the brain has a difficult time analyzing the fullness level in the stomach. Studies have shown that, on average, distracted eating causes people to eat up to 69% more than they normally would.

The key to avoiding this is to be mindful of the things you're doing, especially when it comes to your food intake. Eating slowly and being aware of all the tastes and experience of your food is a good way to start.

Make eating time its own time. Don't eat distracted.

PART 2
NUTRITION LAWS

"Let food be thy medicine, and medicine be thy food"

—HIPPOCRATES

WHEN IT COMES to changing your body composition, nothing is more important than your nutrition. I don't care if you work out three hours a day; if you overeat, you will gain fat. You'll be better off pulling back on your training and dialing in your nutrition and making sure you're eating in a calorie deficit.

For years, I made this mistake. I would try to offset my bad eating by doing more cardio and training. I was making things worse because all I was doing was creating more hunger through increased activity, so I would end up overeating again. This rollercoaster went on for years.

It's better to workout 3-4 days per week for an hour each day and hit your calorie targets instead of training three hours per day, seven days a week and overeating. Eat smart and you won't have to kill yourself in the gym to compensate.

MASTER THE CALORIE GAME

A WHILE BACK, I was approached by the CEO of a Fortune 500 Company to get him into shape. His name was Michael and he was about 50 pounds overweight. He was recommended to me through another one of my clients, Bill. Michael's days were crazy, with meetings from 6 am until midnight almost every day. On top of that, he was traveling every single week. He'd been trying to lose weight for years and he even worked out with a trainer three times per week, but it wasn't enough because his diet was terrible. Michael was a very straight-forward no-BS type of guy.

On our first introductory call, he asked me an important question: "Stephen, can you give me the exact same plan you gave Bill? (Bill dropped 30 lbs in 12 weeks). I just want to lose 50 pounds in the fastest and easiest way possible. I will do whatever you tell me to do. So, can you help me?"

After a series of questions, I realized exactly what his problem was. Like most people, he was eating way too much. I asked him to track his calories the following day. I told him to download the app, MyFitnessPal, on his phone and, to the best of his ability, start tracking how much he ate. The next day we talked again. He was eating around 3800 calories per day. Tons of sweets, and highly processed junk. He needed to be eating around 2200 calories per day to lose fat. So I put him on a nutrition plan and gave him a training program to follow. Each week he sent me his updated weight and photos. In 30 days, he was down 16 pounds. Why? Because he was meticulous about tracking his calories.

Dropping body fat comes down to one thing: BURNING MORE CALORIES THAN YOU CONSUME. This is called creating a CALORIE DEFICIT.

How do you know if you're in a calorie deficit? You need to track your calories.

Here are the two most important things you need to track if you want to get above average results in the fastest time.

1. You must create an appropriate caloric deficit. The easiest way to figure this out is to take your current body weight and multiply it by 12. For example, if your current weight is 200 pounds, then your calorie intake would be: 200 X 12 = 2200 calories per day. That's it. If you follow this simple formula, fat loss will be inevitable.

2. Get enough protein. (0.8g - 1.2g of protein per lb of bodyweight)

For simplicity reasons, I like to multiply body weight by 1. For example, if your current body weight is 200 pounds, then your protein intake would be: 200 X 1 = 200 grams of protein per day. Getting enough protein will ensure you are building/maintaining muscle while dropping body fat.

Think about it this way. A calorie deficit is responsible for **starving the fat**. Eating enough protein is responsible for **feeding the muscle**.

Don't worry about tracking fats and carbs. They are just energy sources, so if you prefer a higher-fat diet, then eat more fats. If you enjoy carbs more, eat more carbs. Again, as long as you are eating in a calorie deficit, you will burn fat.

The only way to force the body to burn stored energy (e.g., body fat) is to create an imbalance between energy intake and energy expenditure. Want to know what all diets (paleo, Keto, low fat, carnivore, Adkins, intermittent fasting) have in common? They all create a calorie deficit.

Now, someone will probably point to someone who lost weight without 'counting calories,' but invariably, they did something dietarily that resulted in them burning more calories than they consumed. They just did it in a way that looked 'different' than simply counting calories. But in the end, the result was the same. They still created a caloric deficit, but it was 'hidden' by what looked like something else (Keto, carb cycling, taking thyroid medication, running 6x per week, etc.).

Download the app, MYFITNESSPAL, right now. It's free. This is the same app I have all of my clients use. I have been using this app every single day for the past five years. It takes me under two minutes a day to track all my calories. Tracking your calories each day will also keep you accountable.

You will also want to buy a food scale. You can get one on Amazon or at Walmart for around $10. Weigh out things like meat, rice, potatoes, oatmeal, etc. Once you have the correct weight, just enter it into MyFitnessPal and boom, done.

LAW #24
PUMP UP YOUR PROTEIN

MOST PEOPLE THINK that protein's main job is to help build muscle, but that is only half true. Protein is just as important for burning fat as it is for building muscle. Out of all the three macronutrients—proteins, carbs, and fats—protein is the most thermogenic macronutrient.

This means your body needs to use more energy to digest and break down protein. Your body burns more calories to digest protein than it does for fats and carbs. For every 100 calories of protein you consume, your body burns 25 - 30 of those calories just for digestion. This is why eating a higher protein diet is critical if fat loss is the goal.

The best way to get your protein will always be to consume whole foods like lean meats, eggs, greek yogurt, etc. If you're having a hard time eating enough food to reach your protein target, then using whey protein powder is very beneficial.

Most protein powders have 25 grams of protein per serving. So, if you have one or two scoops of protein powder with your meals, this is an easy way to get an additional 25 - 50 grams of protein per meal. You can also drink protein shakes between meals or when you are on the go.

LAW #25
RESTRICT YOUR FEEDING WINDOW

FROM THE SECOND I took my first breath, I was taught the importance of religion. Now I'm not here to debate with you who's right or wrong (I'm right). I'm here to provide you with one of the most effortless ways to get abs so defined they have lickable crevices.

Ironically, it originates deep within the traditions of my religion.

In the late 1990's the Mediterranean diet became all the rage because the research suggested that the diet of the Mediterranean region (the island of Crete, Greece) was superior to the Western world's diet.

The Mediterranean diet created a population, on average, that had less heart disease and healthier overall than North Americans.

This theory, while making sense, was missing a key component of the Mediterranean lifestyle: fasting. In the Greek Orthodox Christian Church, there are some very lengthy fasting traditions (around 200 days of the year requires some form of dietary restriction.)

Hundreds of research papers and books later, I learned that short-term (12 hours - 3 days) intermittent fasting, was not only an effective and easy way to cut calories (a fundamental to six pack abs), but was also associated with an array of amazing health benefits including:

- Increased insulin sensitivity
- Increased lipolysis (fat breakdown)
- Increased growth hormone
- Muscle protection
- Effortless abs
- Heightened mental clarity
- Enhanced energy and focus

Intermittent fasting is not a way of telling you what to eat, but a system of telling yourself when to eat.

The window starts when you first ingest something that isn't toothpaste and ends when you have your last bite or sip of beverage that isn't water. It can range from 12 hours - 3 days. My two favorite ways that I would recommend for effectiveness and flexibility are:

1. 24-HOUR FASTS

From the last time you consume a calorie on the previous day to the same time the next day, you will fast, meaning you will consume 0 calories. Black coffee, green tea, lemon water and diet soda are all acceptable.

So for example, if your last meal were at 8 pm the night before, you would start eating at 8 pm the next day.

You would break your fast with a normal, slightly oversized meal full of fresh vegetables, high-quality protein, carbs, and fat. Again, it's the calorie count that matters here (for six pack purposes)

2. 12-18 HOUR FASTS

These will occur daily and depending on how you feel, how busy you are and when you can eat, you will be doing a 12 - 18 hour fast. So if you sleep for on average about 8 hours a night and you stop eating 1-2 hours before bed, you would wake up and push your first meal of the day (commonly known as breakfast) back 4-6 hours.

If you wake up at 7 am, and you stopped eating at ten the night before, then your first meal would be between 10 am and 2 pm. Personally, I break my fast between 12 and 2 pm as that is what works for me and my schedule.

Try it, and watch the magic unfold.

LAW #26
STAY FLEXIBLE

I **F I WERE** to tell you that you can't have any pizza for the next 12 weeks, what is the only food you would obsess over? Pizza, of course. It's human nature. We want what we can't have. This is why most diets fail. They are over-restrictive. When people feel restricted, it's only a matter of time before they break and give in to their cravings and desires.

Most diets today are built around eliminating entire food groups. The Keto diet eliminates all carbs. The carnivore diet eliminates everything besides meat; you can't even have veggies for God's sake. These diets have their place, and I know people with autoimmune issues that have used an elimination diet like Keto and carnivore to treat symptoms of inflammation and gluten sensitivities. However, for 99% of us, these diets are not sustainable.

This is why I believe in taking a flexible approach to your nutrition. Flexible dieting is about having your cake and eating it too. I have many clients who've gotten shredded without giving up any of their favorite foods. My client Amy has two glasses of wine every night, and she has better abs than most lean men. If you're going to be busting your ass in the gym and want to be fit and sexy and sustain it, then you need to find a plan that is sustainable for the rest of your life. Balance is critical.

Just remember this: long-term consistency trumps short-term intensity. The longer you can be consistent with a nutrition plan, the more success you will have. Now, just to be clear, just because you can still enjoy the foods you love, doesn't mean you can eat as much of it as you want. You still need to stay within your daily calorie goal. 80% of the foods you eat should be whole, healthy foods that will fuel your body and keep you full. The other 20% of foods can be what you want. Everything in moderation.

Here is what a typical day might look like for someone who has a calorie goal of 2,000 calories per day:

12 pm (first meal) - 10-ounce ribeye with a baked potato and a small salad - 750 calories

4 pm (snack) - A protein bar and an apple - 350 calories

6 pm (dinner) - 10 ounces of salmon with 1 cup rice and mixed veggies - 700 calories

8 pm (nightcap) - 2 glasses of wine - 200 calories

Daily total: 2,000 calories

Having flexibility with your nutrition allows you to eat your calories on your terms. You no longer have to be a slave to your diet. That's what flexible dieting is all about.

THE 20 FOOD RULE

THE FOUNDER OF Apple, Steve Jobs, was known for wearing the exact same thing every day. He always wore a black turtleneck, blue jeans and white New Balance sneakers. The founder of Facebook, Mark Zuckerburg, also wears the same thing every day, a gray t-shirt, and jeans. Both of them explained that the less time they spent on making decisions (like what to wear in the morning) the more brain power they had to make better decisions for the rest of the day. Why is this?

DECISION FATIGUE.

Decision fatigue is the physiological condition where making a decision in the present will reduce your decision-making ability in the future. Many studies have shown that as humans, our ability to make good decisions is finite. Our ability to make a good decision at the beginning of the day is much greater than at the end of the day.

Decision fatigue is the reason why normal people spend money on random things they don't need or buy a delicious but completely unnecessary 1kg bucket of Nutella at the supermarket. It doesn't matter how much discipline or willpower you have. We are all susceptible to decision fatigue.

The more choices you make throughout the day, the harder each one becomes, and eventually, your brain looks for shortcuts, usually in either one or two different ways:

1. You become reckless. You act impulsively instead of expending the energy to first think through the consequences. (Sure, eat half a pie. I trained hard today. I deserve it. What's the problem?)
2. You do nothing. Instead of agonizing over decisions, you avoid everything at all costs. The problem with this is that there are actually repercussions to your actions, even if your action is to do nothing. Not doing anything often creates bigger problems in the long run, but for the moment, it eases the mental strain.

Let's use dinner as an example. If you've had a decision-filled day, chances are you'll say screw it, and order pizza. Your brain gets a much-needed break, but your body and goals take a hit. Having a list of pre-determined foods to stick to makes deciding what you eat effortless. This leads to more compliance and, ultimately, the achievement of your fitness goals.

Now, you're probably thinking, 'Won't I get tired of eating the same meals every day?' My clients and I have been eating 90% of the same meals regularly for a few years now, and I have yet to get bored of them. But that's because I have a few tricks up my sleeve:

1. I do have the occasional all-you-can-eat cheat meal to spice up my life – mostly for the psychological aspect of giving me a mental break. Plus, life's too short to miss out on deep-fried cheesecake.

2. I do modify the flavor of my meals by getting different types of cheese, adding different seasonings, spices, condiments, and changing up the vegetables that I use. You don't need to be too strict about it. If you feel like you're getting tired of the same meal, then take a break for a couple of days. 20 foods, combined with the two previous principles, should provide more than enough variety for, well, a lifetime.

How many different foods do you eat in a given week? 5? 25? 40? If you are like most people, you fall into the 40+ category. And while variety has been called the spice of life, when it comes to getting a six pack, simplicity is the ultimate sophistication. Keeping your diet relatively simple on a daily basis delivers a near bulletproof formula to achieving six pack abs.

These are my top 20 foods:

Protein: Boneless and skinless chicken breast, turkey breast, eggs, burgers, grass-fed steak, and fish.

Carbs: Potatoes, white rice, banana, strawberries, apples, grapes, and oatmeal.

Fats: Peanut butter, almonds, butter (grass-fed), chocolate (dark), cheese, avocado, and coconut milk (unsweetened).

Once you start simplifying your diet, you'll find it's hard to stop. When eating healthily day in and day out, it becomes effortless, and you will notice how great it makes you feel.

So, what I want you to do is pick 2-3 foods that don't make you feel like crap when you eat them. For me, that was chicken breast, avocados, and sweet potatoes. Only eat those foods for one day. Then the next day, add in another food. Then another. Until you find a food that doesn't fit. Keep testing until you find your top

15-20 foods. Then, eat them for the rest of eternity. Just kidding. Once a month, you can cheat a little bit. Have some pizza, ice cream or deep-fried Oreos. Want to binge-eat 322 gummy worms? I understand.

But in general, stick to your top 20 foods. It will do wonders for your energy, health, and body composition.

KEEP A REGULAR EATING SCHEDULE

WHEN IT COMES to working out, your body loves a new stimulus. When it comes to diet, your body thrives on routine.
Your body is made of circadian rhythms. These rhythms affect how you sleep, but more specifically, how you eat. Emerging research is showing us that we are not just what we eat, but when we eat it.

Researchers at the Salk Institute have found that an erratic meal schedule can disrupt the metabolism and is correlated with chronic disease and a faster aging process. On the other hand, "Initial studies on humans have shown that adhering to a consistent meal schedule correlated with greater fat loss, enhanced ability to sleep, increased growth hormone and stabilization of insulin."

Researchers have shown that we don't even need to change the quality of our foods to elicit a positive fat loss response. All we need to do is change the times we eat.

There's no plug-and-play routine that works best for everyone. It's important to make your eating time fit in with your lifestyle. Figure out what works best for you.

Personally, I eat two meals per day (lunch and dinner) with 1-2 snacks. I also have one client who eats one meal per day at 8 pm and another who eats eight mini-meals every two hours or so. They are both shredded and feel amazing. Experiment and see what works for you.

LAW #29
MAKE YOUR FIRST MEAL PERFECT

WHY DO THEY call it breakfast? Because it is the meal that breaks your fast. Whenever you go an extended period without food (8-20 hours), many hormonal changes happen. The late and great strength coach, Charles Poliquin, said, "The first thing you put in your mouth in the morning dictates all neurotransmitters for the whole day." So what we can gather from this is that our first meal sets the tone for the rest of the day.

There have been many studies on this topic. One Harvard study found that children who had a high-carb sugary breakfast made poorer lunch choices when given the option of choosing what to eat. These children also scored 20% lower on IQ tests. This is significant when compared to children who ate a higher protein and fat breakfast.

In human psychology, there is something called priming. Priming is a technique where exposure to one stimulus influences a response to a subsequent stimulus, without conscious guidance or intention.

How does this translate into dropping body fat and getting lean? The first event of the day will prime your day for good or for bad. On many occasions, my clients (and sometimes myself) have chosen to start the day off with a sugary, carb-loaded meal. For example, chocolate chip pancakes with maple syrup. Obviously, not the best choice, but the damage isn't too terrible. However, as the day goes on, it seems like the subsequent meals will get worse and worse, despite the best intentions.

Here's what I've learned: We can prime our bodies, starting with the first meal. If your first meal is healthy and made up of whole healthy foods like lean meats, eggs, avocado, veggies, etc. then your body will crave those foods more throughout the day. On the flip side, if you start your day eating sugary foods, your body will be primed to crave more of those foods later.

Making the first meal of your day perfect ensures that you prime your body properly to win the day. After all, winning each day helps you win the war. Make getting lean effortless by ensuring your first meal of each day is perfect.

LAW #30
PUMP UP THE VOLUME
- FOOD VOLUME

ON THIS JOURNEY to getting lean and sub-10% body fat, you must realize one thing: Your body DOES NOT want you to be lean. Your body's number one job is to keep you alive by any means necessary. Your body doesn't care what you look like, as long as you're alive. This is both a good thing and a bad thing. It is good because we are, well, alive. But this is terrible if your goal is to get super lean. Thousands of years ago, when food was scarce, your body needed to hold onto fat in case there was a famine. This fat is usually referred to as your "survival fat." This is also your stubborn fat. Typically for men, this is the fat on your lower belly, lower back, and love handles. For women, these areas are usually the thighs and butt. We don't live in a hunter-gatherer world anymore and eating less has many benefits. But you don't have to starve yourself to get lean.

A big reason why many people think they're eating very little but can't lose weight is because they think in terms of food quantity and not calorie content.

The most important thing you must do when you are in a calorie deficit is MANAGE YOUR HUNGER. Hunger is normal, and there will be times during this fat-loss journey when you are hungry. What separates the people who will have fat loss success and those who won't is how they deal with and manage hunger.

This is why food choices are critical when you start a fat-loss program. You need to make sure you eat filling, high-volume but low-calorie foods. Let's say for lunch, I decide to have eight ounces of chicken and a sweet potato. This might keep me full for an hour or so. But let's say I have that same eight ounces of chicken, but I put it over a huge bowl of salad (I mean, a really big bowl of salad) and have my sweet potato. The amount of actual food is a lot, and all of that salad is going to take up a large amount of volume in my stomach. The salad itself is only 20 calories, mostly from fiber. So not only will I be physically full, but this will signal to my brain that I have eaten a lot and my hunger signals will subside.

Again, eating low-calorie, high-volume foods is going to be your secret weapon when it comes to staying full while in a calorie deficit.

Here are some examples of low-calorie, high-volume foods that I include in my diet almost every day:

- Salad, lots of salad
- Spaghetti squash (great substitute for pasta)
- Cauliflower (roasted in the oven with garlic. Tastes incredible)
- Cucumbers
- Pickles
- Carrots (roast in the oven with cinnamon and sea salt)
- Fennel
- Celery
- Asparagus
- Broccoli
- Brussels Sprouts
- Peppers

All of these foods are extremely healthy and are high in micronutrients and phytonutrients. The best part is they're very low calorie, so you can eat as much as you want without stress.

This one diet trick alone has literally changed my life. If you are hungry constantly, it will only be a matter of time before you talk yourself into eating everything in your pantry. Plan for hunger and then control it by eating the foods above.

LAW #31

GO GREEN

THE REASON MOST people start eating healthier is because of vanity reasons. They want to look better naked. And the truth is, there is nothing wrong with that. But, what good is it if you look amazing but feel like crap? Not only do I want to look amazing, but more importantly, I want to feel amazing.

Going back to the previous law, we talked about eating high-volume, low-calorie foods. Greens are not only low calorie and high in volume, they're extremely high in micronutrients and phytonutrients. Leafy greens also contain healthy sugar that helps to increase the amount of good bacteria in the gut. This is important for digestion. Remember, having a healthy digestive system is critical when trying to get lean and lose fat. If your body can't absorb vitamins and nutrients properly, you'll have a much harder time reaching your goals.

Scientific studies are actually finding that the more greens we eat, the more strength and muscle gains we make. I guess Popeye was pretty smart, after all. As you will be consuming a higher protein diet when you are trying to build muscle and burn fat, leafy greens and vegetables help the body absorb the protein and amino acids you are consuming. This will greatly help your digestion. Why is this important?

When we consume a higher protein diet, we increase the acidity in the body. This simply means our body produces more acid to digest and break down the protein. Because of this, we need to make sure our bodies are not overly acidic. Everything that enters our body is a step toward a more acidic or less acidic environment. Once you eat a food consisting of acid-forming ingredients, your body will start to release substances in an effort to balance out the acidic food.

On the contrary, if your diet contains a lot more alkaline foods, there's no imbalance created, and thus your body will not have to mobilize resources to re-balance. This is optimal for losing fat and six pack abs.

If you are eating a lot of acidic foods, liek protein and bread, you'll need low acidic foods to balance it out. In particular, green veggies like broccoli, spinach, and kale will be best.

LAW #32

REFEED, DON'T CHEAT (DON'T CONFUSE CLIMATE AND WEATHER)

IF YOU'VE EVER** had to cut calories for a sustained period, you know that it isn't all fun and games. You can get some serious food cravings, be more irritable, tired, and moody. Even worse, as you decrease calories, your body will down-regulate (slow down) your metabolism in an effort to prevent starvation, often stalling your weight loss and creating hormonal issues with leptin (your hunger hormone), testosterone, and cortisol, to name a few. Not to mention, there's also the burden of the psychological stress that comes with prolonged dieting.

Luckily, there's a simple, yet often overlooked way to combat the negatives:

Refeed Days.

Now, these aren't all-out binge days. Instead, they are strategically targeted caloric spikes used to balance your hormones, keep your metabolism running effectively, and help you reach your fat-loss goals faster. Now, let's talk about how to go about an effective refeed day.

The best way to calculate your calories for a refeed day is to use your maintenance calories. This is calculated by taking your body weight X 18. So if you are 200 pounds, it would look like this:

200 X 18 = 3600 calories.

On a refeed day, you won't be losing fat, but you also won't be gaining fat (if done correctly). During the week, you're taking three steps forward and a refeed day will take you one step back, but will have long-term benefits that will help you reach your goals faster. A refeed day's sole purpose is to balance your hormones, boost your metabolic rate, and give you a day to unwind and enjoy more calories and some of the foods you've been depriving yourself of. The problem is that most people treat a refeed day like a cheat day, and they stuff their face for 24 hours with anything and everything. I am going to warn you:

IF YOU TREAT YOUR REFEED DAY LIKE A CHEAT DAY, YOU'VE JUST ELIMINATED ALL YOUR HARD WORK AND PROGRESS FOR THE ENTIRE WEEK.

Yes, you can destroy a week's worth of progress in one day. I have done it more times than I'd like to admit. The sooner you get off of that cheat day roller coaster, the sooner you will have the body you want. It's that simple.

As for what to eat on your refeed day, remember that carbs are king. They provide the biggest boost in metabolism. Carbs replenish muscle glycogen (fuel stored in the muscles) so your workouts following the days after a refeed will be amazing. Your muscles will swell and your muscle pumps will be incredible.

Again, this isn't a full-blown cheat day. It's a planned and structured day of increased calories to help your body burn more fat so you can reach your goals faster.

HOW OFTEN SHOULD YOU INCLUDE A REFEED DAY?

The leaner you are, the more often you can have a refeed day. If you are above 15% body fat, you should only have a refeed day once every two weeks. As your body fat drops, you can increase the frequency of your refeed days. If you are under 15% body fat, you can get away with one refeed day per week. Once you are in the 10-12% body fat range, you can do refeed days 2-3 times per week. Again, the leaner you are, the more often you can incorporate refeed days.

LAW #33
FEAST AT NIGHT

NTERMITTENT FASTING IS a tool I use almost every day for calorie control. It works with my lifestyle because I am usually busy all morning up until late afternoon, so I usually don't have time to eat a big meal. I will sip coffee throughout the morning and early afternoon and I might have a snack if I feel hungry, which usually consists of a protein bar or a protein shake with an apple.

The best feeling in the world is getting home at the end of a long day and still having most of your calories left to eat. This allows me to eat HUGE, delicious meals at night. Let's face it, when you've had a long day, you want to get home, unwind, destress, and enjoy some good food…and maybe a drink…or two. Pushing your calories back later in the day allows you to do just that.

I don't know about you, but the biggest issue I have is sticking to my diet at night. So instead of fighting it, I plan for it. It's that simple. You know yourself better than anyone, so if you know you are more hungry at night, and if you are more likely to give in to temptation at night, you need to make adjustments to your meal timing to avoid overeating.

I recommend you save 50-60% of your daily calories for your evening meal. It's much easier to eat lighter during the day if you know you can look forward to a delicious 1000-calorie feast at night.

It takes a lot of willpower to go to bed hungry. Going to bed hungry can also lead to poor sleep.

So, try this out, save 50-60% of your calories for your evening meal. And don't worry, eating big at night won't make you fat. It's all about the macros and calories. Your body doesn't magically store any food eaten after 8 pm as fat, despite what mainstream diet advice might have you believe.

LAW #34
TAKE A SMOKER'S BREAK AFTER YOU EAT

SMOKER'S HAVE AN uncanny ability to stay lean. One of the reasons, of course, is that cigarette's help suppress hunger. The other reason is that they get fresh air and don't sit as much, because they take smoking breaks every few hours.

Now don't take this the wrong way. I'm not telling you to pick up a smoking habit. However, I am telling you to move more and get fresh oxygen, as much as possible. This is especially true after eating.

The worst thing anyone can do is to sit or lay down after they eat a meal. Research has shown that walking and getting fresh oxygen for ten minutes after eating helps to speed up the time it takes from the food to move from the stomach into the small intestine.

One small study co-authored by Loretta DiPietro, a professor of exercise science at George Washington University's Milken Institute School of Public Health, found that when older adults at risk for type 2 diabetes walked on a treadmill for 15 minutes after a meal, they had smaller blood sugar spikes in the hours afterward. In fact, the researchers found that these short post-meal walks were even more effective at lowering blood sugar after dinner than a single 45-minute walk taken at mid-morning or late in the afternoon.

DiPietro points out that many of us eat our largest meal of the day in the evening, and we also tend to sit around afterward. As a result, "blood glucose levels will rise very high and will stay elevated for hours," she says.

So what good does walking do after eating a meal? "The muscles we use to walk use glucose as energy, drawing it out of circulation and therefore reducing how much is floating around," says Andrew Reynolds, a postdoctoral research fellow at the University of Otago in New Zealand.

Walking after a meal increases insulin sensitivity. This means your body will secrete less of it. Insulin is a storage hormone, so any time your body is able to secrete less insulin, this will benefit you when it comes to getting lean.

Moving and walking after a meal also helps your body to encourage the digestion process along faster. Having more efficient digestion means better overall health.

So, try taking a smokers break and walk for ten minutes after each meal. If you eat three times per day, this could be 30 minutes of walking. This alone can burn an additional 200-300 calories per day.

HAVE AT LEAST FIVE GO-TO MEALS

I DON'T KNOW ABOUT you, but I know what I like, especially when it comes to food. There are certain times when I want to be creative and explore different foods and different restaurants, but for the most part, I go to the same restaurants and cook the same food at home every day, because I like it. When it comes to getting lean and losing body fat, variety is not always beneficial. Keeping things simple and easy will allow you to reach your goal much faster.

I eat mostly the same foods every day because they taste good and I know the nutritional value of them. My dinner for the last two years has been pretty much the same thing: a big salad with a pound of chicken, a whole avocado, tomatoes, cucumbers, and a healthy Greek yogurt dressing I make. This is my 'go-to' meal. I look forward to it every day because it tastes amazing, it's healthy, and it fills me up. I have 3-4 other meals that I rotate throughout the week. These are my top five meals I eat. This way, I don't have to think about what I am going to make when I get home every day.

Go-to meals save you time and reduce the stress and anxiety of what you should eat and how much. Here's what I suggest: have five go-to meals. Two for breakfast (if you aren't fasting), two or three for lunch/dinner, two for when you're on the road and a snack. Here are mine:

Breakfast A: Egg omelet with veggies and protein, plus 2 pieces of toast or 250g oatmeal.

Breakfast B: 1 scoop of whey protein with 1 cup of almond/coconut milk, 1 banana, 1tbsp of peanut butter, 2-3 handfuls of spinach, and some cinnamon.

Lunch A: 16 ounces chicken or salmon in a mixed green salad with one whole avocado, tomatoes, cucumbers, and my Greek dressing.

Lunch B: Turkey or tuna sandwich and a side of greens (or greens drink) and blackberries.

Dinner: 300g of fish, 400g of potatoes and a side salad or green juice.

Snack: 1-2 protein bars or an apple with 1 scoop of powder mixed with water.

Outing 1: Chipotle salad bowl - base salad with double chicken, triple veggie, black beans, half rice, hot salsa, and guacamole.

Outing 2: Steak, salad and baked potato.

The more simplistic you keep things with your nutrition, the better. Figure out what you like, and then create some meals you can rotate into your plan throughout the week.

LAW #36
DESTROY TEMPTATION

WHEN I LIVED at home with my family, reaching my fat-loss goals were extremely difficult. The pantry and fridge were packed with sweets and snacks. Regardless of how hard I tried, it was only a matter of time before I gave into temptation and ate the entire package of Oreos or a whole box of Lucky Charms cereal.

When I moved to Toronto, my roommate was also a fitness guy. We were both trying to get lean, so we decided to eliminate any kind of temptation. No snacks and no sweets. We were so set on reaching our goals that we only bought enough food for each day. So each day I would go to the grocery store, usually after the gym, and I would buy just enough food for that day. Typically I would buy salad, ground meat, and Greek yogurt. We lived about ¼ mile away from the grocery store, so if we did have cravings at night, we literally had to walk ¼ mile to get what we wanted…so as you can guess, we typically didn't go.

If an alcoholic decided they wanted to get sober and change their life, what is the first thing they would do? They would stop going to the bar, and they would throw out any alcohol they had at home. You need to treat your situation the same way. If you are serious about transforming your body and getting lean, you need to destroy any temptation that will keep you from reaching your goals.

The first step to succeeding at pretty much anything in life is to set up your environment for success. The more distractions and roadblocks there are, the harder it's going to be to achieve the outcome you're hoping for. This is especially true when it comes to healthy eating.

Studies show we make about 200 food decisions every day. If your house and workspace are full of food, it will derail your goals, and you're unlikely to win. It can happen to even the most disciplined individuals. As soon as your stress levels reach a certain point, you'll switch to a medication-seeking state.

Our ancestors, thousands of years ago, figured out that when they ate something sweet and tasty, they decreased cortisol (your stress hormone). This is because sugar lights up the brain's reward center. When we eat sugar, the body secretes a hormone called serotonin. Serotonin makes you feel relaxed and happy, so it makes perfect sense that we would want sweet and sugary foods when we're stressed.

If your fridge and pantry are stocked full of "medication" in the form of hyper-palatable comfort foods, it won't be long until you reach for them. On the other hand, if these foods aren't available, you'll have an opportunity to make alternative and better choices.

So, the first step toward improving your short-term success rate is to make changes to your immediate environment. Get rid of everything that doesn't align with your goals. This doesn't mean you'll never eat these foods ever again; it just means that you're not going to keep them "locked and loaded" at all times. Your body and behavior are a reflection of the environment you place yourself in. Minimize temptation proximity and make your environment reflect the goals you've set for yourself.

If you have a family or kids and keep these highly tempting foods in the house, then just tell your spouse to hide them or put them somewhere you won't find them. Whenever I go home and stay with my family for the holidays, I always tell them "hide the peanut butter." I'm not kidding. Peanut butter is a trigger food for me. I can literally sit down and eat an entire container in one sitting. But because I know this about myself, I tell them to hide it so I won't be tempted. Is this too extreme? Maybe. But I am extreme when it comes to reaching my goals, and you should be too.

LAW #37
AVOID GETTING DRUNK

I HAVE NEVER BEEN a big drinker. When I go on a date or out with friends, I will usually have a few beers with dinner or a glass of wine, but I was never the party animal who drank until the point of passing out. I would much rather eat my calories than drink them, but this is not the case for everyone, and I have many clients who drink, some drink daily, but in moderation.

Alcohol has a unique association with an increased waistline. But it's not necessarily what you think. As we know, to get lean, we need to burn more energy than we consume.

Alcohol is calorically dense, packing 7 calories per gram. If your main objective is to get lean and reach your physique goals, then you should cut back or preferably halt consumption altogether, especially if alcohol is a trigger for you.

Beer can range from 60 to 250 calories per serving; one shot of liquor contains up to 200 calories, and when you're tossing that into a sugary fruit juice or soda, you're looking at hundreds of calories per drink. Alcohol can also mess up your gut biome and delicate hormonal balance, which doesn't help either. Now, it's possible to enjoy alcohol and still get ripped. However, alcohol, like many drugs, has another sinister effect on the body: poor decision-making.

Often, after coming home from the bar, people turn to greasy food for comfort. In a sober state, aligned with your goals, you would turn down the 2000-calorie pepperoni pizza. Alcohol sabotages you into rationalizing this behavior, often resulting in 2000-calorie binges (I've done this too many times to count). These mini-binges absolutely destroy any chance of having abs.

Avoiding (or limiting) alcohol is a key component when trying to achieve a low level of body fat. That being said, once you've gotten there, it's much easier to throw back a few and still keep your abs. Everything in moderation.

LAW #38
DON'T DRINK YOUR CALORIES

A **FEW YEARS BACK,** I was working with a client named Al. Al was addicted to soda. He would drink 4-5 cokes per day. That's 800-1000 calories of soda per day. The first week we started working together; I didn't change his diet or have him work out. I asked him to do one thing - start drinking diet coke instead of regular coke. He did it, and he dropped six pounds that first week.

One of the most common weight loss mistakes I see people making is drinking their calories. The major problem with caloric beverages like soda, sports and energy drinks, and fruit juices, is that they don't trigger satiety like food does.

You can drink 1,000 calories and be hungry an hour later, whereas eating 1,000 calories of food, including a good portion of protein and fiber, will probably keep you full for five to six hours. The volume food takes up in your stomach compared to liquids isn't even close.

Researchers from Purdue University, who investigated the influence of meal timing and food form on daily energy intake found this: "Based on the appetitive findings, consumption of an energy-yielding beverage either with a meal or as a snack poses a greater risk for promoting positive energy than macronutrient-matched semisolid or solid foods consumed at these times." That is, people that drink calories are much more likely to overeat than those who don't. This is why research shows a clear association between greater intakes of sugar-sweetened beverages and weight gain in both adults and children.

So, ditch the high-calorie beverages and opt for water, seltzer, or naturally sweetened zero-calorie alternatives instead.

LAW #39
GET HYDRATED

EVERYONE ACCEPTS THAT water is essential for life, yet hardly anyone drinks enough of the stuff. Studies show that 75% of the population is dehydrated, leading to many different metabolic disruptions, most of which affect your ability to get lean.

Once your kidneys become dehydrated, their main job of filtering the blood becomes inhibited, and this passes a lot of the workload onto the liver. One of your liver's main functions is to metabolize stored body fat. If your kidneys are malfunctioning from dehydration, then your liver can't do its job effectively.

Human Growth hormone (HGH), a potent fat-burning hormone, is greatly reduced when the body is dehydrated, limiting fat metabolism. Even the enzyme that metabolizes fat, Lipase, has significantly reduced function when the body isn't fully hydrated.

Another issue with dehydration is how it affects the brain. The brain is made of roughly 80% water and is therefore very sensitive to changes in water levels. Just 2% dehydration can reduce cognitive function by up to 30%. This leads to false tiredness, low motivation and a lack of willpower (often the main culprits for derailing any chances of getting lean). Dehydration is also tricky because it's easy to confuse the symptoms with other things. You can go crazy trying to figure out what's wrong without realizing it all stems from simply not drinking enough water. So, then, how much water should you be drinking exactly?

If you start with a baseline water intake of about 3/4 to 1 gallon per day, you will be good. Personally, I'll drink one liter as soon as I wake up and then sip on a few bottles throughout the day. If my pee isn't clear, I'm not drinking enough. One thing to note: not all water is created equal.

Research shows that standard tap water is becoming more and more contaminated with all kinds of pollutants, including bacteria, pharmaceuticals, heavy metals, and various types of poisonous chemicals. Bottled water isn't much better. One study examined 18 different bottled waters from 13 different companies and found over 24,000 chemicals present, including endocrine disruptors. This is why I recommend (and personally drink) distilled water or reverse osmosis water. If it is out of your budget, filtered tap water is just fine.

BUY SINGLE SERVINGS

OVER THE YEARS, I've had many clients that did amazing during the day their nutrition and training, but at night, they would fall into temptation, give in to their weakness, and binge on a pint of ice cream (or other junk food) and destroy their progress. Even when I allowed them to eat a little bit of ice cream, they would still end up having a major binge episode. Here's what I've found: People are wired to eat until the food is done, not until they feel satisfied.

Have you ever noticed how easy it is to overeat ice cream, chips, cookies, cookies, or any food that comes in a bag, box, or container? When the food is available, and it's in front of us, we have to make a real effort to stop. But what if you only had the quantity you planned to eat? Or a quantity that wouldn't completely destroy your progress? You wouldn't have to use any willpower. Even if you wanted to eat more, you wouldn't be able to.

That's why I often prescribe single-serving purchases to my clients. Having one ice cream bar in the house as opposed to a pint of ice cream means that once the bar is done, no matter how badly you want more, you can't overeat. That's how you make success automatic. You need to set specific restrictions and have safeguards in place to avoid falling off track.

The solution? Don't bring large amounts of binge-worthy foods into the house. Only buy single servings or individually packed servings. Individually packaged servings give you a chance to ask yourself if you really need to keep eating. I've found that most of the time, it'll be enough to make you stop.

Overeating by 300 calories won't hurt you. But binging 1,000+ calories will. So, limit the amount of damage you can do by limiting the amount of food you have. Buy single servings.

DRINK THE SIX PACK SHAKE

WHAT YOU EAT — carbs, fat, protein, some combination thereof, or nothing at all — determines your body's reaction to food and training for the rest of that day. Getting lean, staying lean, and adding muscle, therefore, requires doing things right, and that includes starting the day with a single goal: keep the body burning fat for as long as possible.

The majority of my clients (as well as myself), delay eating breakfast by a few hours for this goal—the easiest solution. I often get up at 6 a.m., but if I eat breakfast, it won't be until 11 am or later —sometimes much later—around 2 pm.

That's a long gap to go without anything—most people need something to curb their appetite, which may be pretty strong in the morning due to the release of the hunger-stimulating hormone ghrelin.

Which is why we created the six pack shake.

Designed to turn your metabolism into a calorie burning inferno that incinerates belly fat, it's one of the most useful tools in our arsenal. And with a little science, we took it a bit further, adding a few ingredients that help turn your metabolism into a calorie burning inferno that incinerates belly fat on demand.

Goal	Ingredient	Amount
Control Hunger & Accelerate Fat Mobilization	Black coffee (decaf or regular)	1-2 Cups (hot or cold)
Protect Muscle Breakdown & Crush hunger	100% Whey Isolate Or Vegan Protein Powder	10g or ⅓ of a scoop
Prolong Ketogenesis & Improve focus	Coconut milk & MCTs	½ - 1 Cup of coconut milk + 1bsp of MCT oil/ powder (optional)
Proper adrenal functioning & Electrolyte Balance	Pink Himilayan Sea Salt	A Pinch
Improve insulin sensitivity & Flavor	Cinnamon	A Pinch
Powerful Antioxidants & Flavor	Raw cacao powder	A Pinch
Satisfy sugar cravings (optional)	Stevia	As much as desired

Directions: Take all ingredients and blend until creamy. Feel free to top with cinnamon, salt and raw cocoa powder instead of blending them in. Consume hot or cold, to break your fast, or as your first "meal" every day.

PART 3
TRAINING LAWS

"Pain makes me grow, growing is what I want. Therefore, for me, pain is pleasure."

—Arnold Schwarzenegger

ONCE YOU HAVE your nutrition dialed in, training will accelerate your results. The goal when it comes to training is to gain lean muscle while burning fat. This is why doing too much cardio won't help you.

Cardio burns calories, but only doing cardio will leave you with loose skin and a skinny-fat physique. This is what we want to avoid. If you go from fat to skinny-fat, what did you really achieve?

The objective is to look like a real-life superhero and create an athletic and fit-looking physique. This is only possible with weight training.

Let's jump into the laws of training.

LAW #42
FOCUS ON BUILDING MUSCLE

LET ME ASK you a question. If I told you there was a way you could burn more calories each day by doing absolutely nothing, would you want to know how? Of course, you would. Here's the secret. Increase the amount of muscle tissue on your body.

Muscle tissue is metabolically active. This simply means that muscles require a significant amount of oxygen and nutrients. This is good news for you because the more muscle you have on your frame, the more energy your body uses to support this muscle mass. When your body uses more energy, you burn more calories.

Christopher Wharton, PhD, a certified personal trainer and researcher with the Rudd Center for Food Policy and Obesity at Yale University says, "10 pounds of muscle burns about 50 calories at rest."

This is why professional bodybuilders need to eat so much. They need to maintain their muscle mass. They are essentially fat-burning machines because of the amount of muscle they have on their frames.

METABOLIC RESISTANCE TRAINING (MRT)

MRT IS THE combination of cardio and weights. Some would classify this type of training as HIIT (High-Intensity Interval Training).

The objective of this style of training is to do two things:

1. Spend less time in the gym.
2. Burn as many calories as possible in the shortest amount of time.

We have all seen that one guy at the gym. He's sitting on the bench press playing on his phone for five minutes, then he does a set and plays on his phone for another ten minutes. A set that should last no more than five minutes ends up lasting 20 minutes, and nothing is accomplished.

The idea with MRT is to get in and get out and cause as much muscle damage as possible. Typically the best way to do this is through supersets.

A superset is performing one exercise and then immediately performing another exercise.

For example:

You do one set of bench presses. You rack the weight and immediately grab the curl bar and start doing bicep curls. There is no rest between these movements. That would be considered one superset. You would rest 60-90 seconds at most and then do another superset.

Training this way serves two purposes:

1. You are breaking down muscle but utilizing weight training.
2. You are decreasing your rest time, which means you're increasing your heart rate and therefore burning more calories.

This is the style of training I have used for years to build muscle and burn fat. Minimizing your rest periods will ensure you're in a fat-burning state throughout your workout.

When you train this way, you will not be able to go more than 60 minutes because your body will be completely depleted. If you are able to train more than 60 minutes, you are not training with enough intensity. Shorten your rest periods.

LAW #44
STRENGTHEN YOUR NEURAL-ABDOMINAL CONNECTION

HAVE YOU EVER tried to work your abs, but you only feel your hip flexors working instead?

This is due to a poor neural-abdominal connection. Without fixing this, no matter how lean you get or how many crunches you do, you'll always fall short of achieving that coveted, chiseled six pack.

Let's banish that for good with some good ol' fashioned Neural Abdominal Reprogramming. The goal is to radically enhance your ability to recruit your abdominal muscles. To stimulate your abs, you need to be good at contracting them voluntarily.

As such, we'll use the lowest skill and least-demanding exercise in the program. Once you get the hang of it, you want to challenge yourself. It's very important that you try to make these exercises hard.

The way you do this is simple: Flex your abs as hard as humanly possible for every second of the exercise, while completing the exercise. You want to squeeze your abs almost as if you are about to get punched in the stomach. Think about how hard you would contract and squeeze your abs.

Every session will use the same ab exercises because the repetition helps improve your capacity to activate your abdominals. Progress will be measured by improving your neuro-abdominal connection: how hard and long you can flex your abs from session to session, week to week. Since most of these movements are free of weights, how difficult they feel will depend on how good you are at tensing your abs. If you can do more than 15 reps of a bodyweight abs exercise, you are not squeezing hard enough. Remember, the goal isn't reps, it's tension.

For the below ab workout, do what it takes to fail in the prescribed time zone (don't worry about the reps).

Exercise	Time	Sets	Rest
Weighted hanging leg raises	30-60s	3-4	1 minute
Weighted incline crunch	30-60s	3-4	1 minute
Weighted cable crunch	30-60s	3-4	1 minute
Russian twist with medicine ball	30-60s	3-4	1 minute

LAW #45
START WITH COMPOUND MOVEMENTS

A COMPOUND EXERCISE IS an exercise that requires multiple muscle groups to work at the same time. For example, squats work the hamstrings, quads, glutes, and calves. Another example would be deadlifts. Deadlifts work the legs, back, and biceps. Because compound exercises involve working more muscles, you are burning more calories to move the weight.

Compound exercises require a lot of energy, so I like to start my workout with compound movements first, when I am at my strongest and then move on to more isolation exercises. Here is what an example training split of mine looks like using compound lifts:

Day 1: Chest/ Triceps – Start with Bench Press
Day 2: Back/Biceps – Start with Deadlifts
Day 3: Legs – Start with Squats
Day 4: Shoulders – Start with Dumbbell or Barbell Press

Always start your workout with a compound lift when you are at your strongest.

LAW #46
TRAIN FASTED

SOME PEOPLE SWEAR by fasted training, and others say it's ineffective and harmful. Well, both are right. It's effective if you do it right and harmful if you do it wrong. Right off the bat, I will say that 99% of the time, I train fasted. And you should too, mainly because it accelerates fat loss, specifically stubborn fat which, in men, is the fat covering your abs and the fat on your lower back (love handles).

Let's get one thing straight, "fasted" training is NOT simply training on an "empty stomach." When your body is digesting, it is in a "fed" or "postprandial" state (prandial means "having to do with a meal"). Once it has finished absorbing the nutrients, your insulin levels drop to a "minimum" (or "baseline" level), and you enter a "fasted" or "postabsorptive" state.

Every day, your body shifts between "fed" and "fasted." When your body is in a fed state, it can't burn fat. Thus, training in a fasted state allows us to accelerate "real" fat loss.

But here's the real magic, training fasted specifically helps to accelerate the burning of stubborn fat. The reason is that fasted training increases blood flow to those problem areas, allowing the fat to be released and mobilized into the bloodstream and finally burned off.

Think about it this way: food is fuel. If you eat a meal and then go to the gym, your body is going to use the food in your belly as fuel. On the flip side, if you wake up and workout without eating, your body doesn't have an immediate fuel source (food) to use for energy, so your body is going to use your stored body fat as an energy source. This is why training fasted is so effective for fat loss.

LAW #47
ELIMINATE DISTRACTIONS

DISTRACTIONS ARE EVERYWHERE, especially in the gym. This is why having a plan is critical. Your workout should start before you even get to the gym. You should already know what workout and what exercises you're doing that day.

Create a training schedule for yourself so you know exactly what you're training and what day you're training it.

For example:
> Monday - Chest/arms
> Tuesday - Back/shoulders
> Wednesday - Legs
> Thursday - Rest
> Friday - Chest/arms
> Saturday - Back/shoulders
> Sunday - Rest

Another thing I do to eliminate distractions is to put my music on. As most of us use our phones for music, I always turn airplane mode on as soon as I get in the gym. Any texts, calls, emails, or social media notifications can wait until I'm finished. This time spent in the gym serves one purpose and one purpose only: to get you closer to your goal. As soon as my headphones go on, it's my time to completely focus on myself and my training. Nothing else matters for the next 45-60 minutes.

LAW #48
WORK ON YOUR WHEELS

NO, I'M NOT talking about your car. You need to train your legs. Your legs are 70-80% of your body's total muscle mass. So, it makes sense that training them would require more energy and burn more calories.

Working bigger muscle groups, like legs, requires your heart and brain to work harder, therefore increasing metabolism.

Weight training is critical for fat loss because of the "after-burn" effect. The after-burn effect simply means that your body is burning calories and using energy for up to 72 hours after the workout is over, to help repair, recover and rebuild the muscle you just broke down in the gym. As 70-80% of your body's muscle mass is in your legs, the after-burn effect after training legs is significantly higher than if you were to train a smaller muscle group.

USE PROGRESSIVE OVERLOAD

DURING THE 6TH century, there was a wrestler called Milo from the Greek city of Croton. Milo is most known for his training. He would lift a baby calf every day until it eventually grew into an adult bull. As Milo did this every day; he eventually got stronger and bigger as the calf grew.

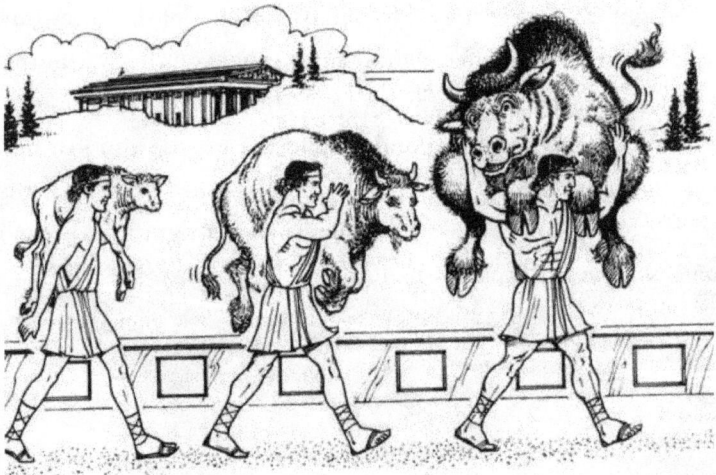

The way you build muscle is by overloading it with stress (weight). This is called Progressive Overload. When you lift weights, your muscles are forced to adapt to the stimulus by getting bigger and stronger. If you aren't continuously challenging your muscles, you will plateau, and results will stop.

The way we continue to grow and make progress is by pushing our bodies harder than we did the time before. Every time you step in the gym, your goal should be to add a little bit more weight. If you can't add more weight, then try to squeeze out one or two more reps.

DON'T OVERDO THE CARDIO

A **WHILE BACK, I** worked with a marathon runner named James. James was trying to drop the last little bit of fat to help improve his race time. As you can imagine, his daily running logs were pretty high. The reason he came to me was, despite dropping his calories and running more, he couldn't lose any weight. In fact, he had actually put on weight.

When we started working together, I gave him two options: to decrease his activity and run less OR increase his calories. He adamantly refused; how could that possibly work? I tried to point out that what he was doing wasn't working, and he had nothing to lose by trying something different, but it didn't matter. He fought me on it and wouldn't do it.

Well, James decided to take his family on vacation. He did what everyone did on vacation; he exercised less and ate more. He came back about five pounds lighter. I remember telling him, "See, you ate more and exercised less, and good things happened."

Over the next several weeks, we increased his calories slowly. His body fat (as measured by DEXA) went from 13.2% to 11.5%, and his metabolic rate increased. He lost the remaining fat almost effortlessly, and he destroyed his race times.

So what the hell was going on? Here's what the research says.

Whenever you are in a severe calorie deficit, and you have a high activity level (especially higher-intensity activity), your metabolism will down-regulate (slow down). Remember, your body doesn't want you to be lean and shredded; it only wants to keep you alive. When you severely restrict calories and increase your activity, your body essentially thinks you're dying and does everything it can to fight back and hold onto your survival fat. Your body does this by slowing down your metabolism so you burn fewer and fewer calories regardless of how little you eat and how much activity you do.

It's not always as simple as calories in, calories out.

Also, when you do excessive cardio (as prescribed by many trainers), you end up not being able to stick to a diet. Excessive cardio pumps up your hunger hormones, making it difficult to stick to an already restrictive diet.

If your car was sitting in your driveway all the time, how much gas would it need? None. It's not moving, so there's no need to fuel it. Now, if you want to go on a road trip, how much gas will your car need? A lot. The more you drive your car, the more fuel it's going to require.

The human body is the same way. The more you move, and the more you exercise, the more energy you're burning and your body is going to require more fuel (food). Activity increases hunger.

I made this mistake for years. I would binge eat one day and then try to make up for it the next few days by doing hours of cardio and eating very little. All I was doing was creating more hunger and more cravings. So I would end up binging again a day or two later. I was creating my own problem by increasing my hunger.

One of my fitness coaches taught me very early on, "you will be much better off doing less cardio and putting less stress on your body and just be more consistent with your nutrition. If you can be more consistent with your nutrition, you won't have to kill yourself by doing tons of cardio." This taught me one thing: work smarter, not harder.

If you find yourself having to do tons of cardio to lose weight, then your activity is not the problem. Something is broken with your nutrition. Fix your nutrition first, and you will set yourself up for success in the long term.

Here's my six pack cardio prescription:
Perform up to 25 minutes of cardio 3x/week maximum. You can do this after or before weight training or on your rest days. If you want to add more cardio, start walking for 30 min-1 hour per day. Walking is low-impact, it burns a lot of calories, and it helps increase blood flow, which helps with recovery.

LAW #51
STAND UP

SITTING IS THE NEW SMOKING.

WHEN YOU SIT for lengthy periods, you alter your body's metabolism. Gavin Bradley, director of Active Working, says, "metabolism slows down 90 percent after 30 minutes of sitting. The enzymes that move the bad fat from your arteries to your muscles, where it can get burned off, slow down. The muscles in your lower body are turned off. And after two hours, good cholesterol drops 20 percent. Just getting up for five minutes is going to get things going again. These things are so simple they're almost stupid."

Toni Yancey, a professor of health services at UCLA's Fielding School of Public Health, describes the process: "Sitting shuts down electrical activity in the legs. It makes the body less sensitive to insulin, causes calorie-burning to plummet, and slows the breakdown of dangerous blood fats, lowering 'good' HDL cholesterol."

How many hours do you sit per day? Global studies show that, on average, we sit for 7.7 hours per day, and some studies estimate people sit for up to 15 hours per day. Don't believe me? Think about it. You sit for three meals, on your way to work, at work, on your way home, and most likely in front of the TV at night. That's a lot of sitting.

Sitting is a silent killer that sneaks up on you, even if you're healthy. Not only does sitting promote aches, pains, cancer, and obesity, but chronic sitting actually makes it almost impossible to achieve a six pack. Why? Because sitting dramatically lowers your body's ability to burn stored energy, silently sabotaging your six pack quest. There's a simple solution, though. Stand as much as possible.

If you just switched to a standing desk at work (eight hours per day), you would burn an extra 200-400 calories. It doesn't seem like that much over a day, but within a year, that's about 31 lbs of fat burned. That is, on average, the amount of fat people need to lose to get within striking distance of their six pack. Just stand.

Katy Bowman, a scientist and author of the book: Move Your DNA: Restore Your Health Through Natural Movement, told Reuters: "You can't offset 10 hours of stillness with one hour of exercise."

LAW #52
WALK IT OUT

T'S NO SECRET, the more you move, the more calories you burn. The amount you walk plays a big role in how much weight you lose and how fast you will lose it. Walking for only 30 minutes can burn up to 200 calories.

Here are some simple ways you can start walking more:
- Take your dog for a walk
- Walk while you are on a phone call
- Park farther away from the store
- Put on a podcast or music while you walk
- Take the stairs whenever you can

The more you move, the more calories you will burn. It's that simple.

MAKE IT BURN

WE'VE ALL SEEN it before. That one guy at the gym who is yelling like a maniac as he does barbell curls with form so terrible that his lower back is doing 90% of the work. Unfortunately, this is how many guys train. They just throw heavy weights around without focusing on the actual muscle they are working. If you want to build muscle, and I'm assuming you do, then you need to maximize your sets by focusing on the muscle you're working.

We do this by utilizing Time Under Tension (TUT). TUT refers to the amount of time a muscle is under stress during the set. For example: You do ten reps of barbell bench presses, taking about one second to press the weight up and 2-3 seconds to lower it back down to your chest.

The most effective way to use TUT correctly is by controlling the negative. The first part of the lift should always be explosive. Using the bench press as an example, you should press the bar as hard as you can, but on the negative (lowering the bar), you want to have maximum control by slowing the descent of the bar back down to your chest. In your head, you should count 2-3 seconds. You don't want to just bounce the bar off your chest because you will be missing out on some serious gains.

Another exercise example is the Barbell Bicep Curl. If you were doing bicep curls, you would curl the bar up and slowly lower the bar for 2-3 seconds.

Again, the purpose of using TUT is to overload the muscle for as long as possible. So the longer the muscle is overloaded, the better. Oh…and yes…it will burn…but that's how you know it's working.

PART 4
REST & RECOVERY LAWS

"Sleep is extremely important to me - I need to rest and recover in order for the training I do to be absorbed by my body"

—*USAIN BOLT*

CONTRARY TO WHAT most people think, you're not growing in the gym. You grow when you sleep. The time spent in the gym is meant to break down muscle and create micro-tears in the muscle fibers. These fibers then heal and grow back bigger and stronger. If you don't allow your body time to get proper rest and recovery, then you will never reap the benefits of your training.

It's critical that you prioritize your rest days. I suggest resting two days per week. You can do some light activity to burn calories like walking, biking, sports, cardio...but no weights. If you are truly training hard for five days per week, then you MUST take these days off to let your body recover.

One of the most important things when it comes to recovery is your nutrition and sleep. We have already covered nutrition, so in this section, we will cover how you can get the most out of your sleep.

LAW #54

PLAN YOUR RECOVERY

MAGINE YOU WERE eating high-quality, healthy, whole foods high in micronutrients, phytonutrients, vitamins, and minerals. Every time you ate these foods, you had to run to the bathroom, and your body couldn't digest or absorb all the nutrients you were eating. Then eating all of this amazing healthy nutrient-dense food wouldn't benefit you in any way, right?

This is how you need to think about your recovery and rest days. Most people don't give their bodies enough time to actually absorb the training they are doing. When they go to the gym, they aren't fully recovered from the previous day, and they're actually doing more harm than good. Your muscles need the rest, but your Central Nervous System (CNS) also needs rest and recovery. Whenever you're training hard and heavy, you tax your CNS, so it's important to properly recover.

I will be honest, taking a rest day is hard for me because I'm addicted to training. My body craves it. So I need to be intentional about taking a rest day away from the weights.

It's important to repeat this: you are NOT building muscle in the gym. You build muscle when you're resting and recovering.

Now, this doesn't mean that you can't do any activity on your rest days. I personally like to do something called Active Recovery. Active recovery involves things like cardio, mobility, flexibility and injury-proofing type movements. You can ride a bike, walk, do yoga, play sports, stretch…anything that doesn't involve using heavy weights.

Here is what my typical training week looks like:

Monday - Weights

Tuesday - Weights

Wednesday - Active Recovery

Thursday - Weights

Friday - Weights

Saturday - Active Recovery

Sunday - Rest (no activity)

Figure out the best schedule for you. Weight training 4-5 days per week is more than enough if you are training hard. Be intentional about your rest days and give your body the rest it needs.

LAW #55

SLEEP DEEP, SLEEP LONG, AND SLEEP MORE

FEELING UNDERSLEPT? **68** million Americans are. But a bad night's sleep doesn't just make for an awful morning. It makes for an awful week. Month. Year. And the impact on our health is far more negative than we might think.

Insufficient sleep has been connected to car crashes, industrial disasters, and other occupational mistakes. It increases the mortality and risk of chronic diseases like hypertension, diabetes, depression, low testosterone, obesity, cancer, and it decreases quality of life.

Inadequate sleep can specifically cause belly fat storage, silently destroying your chances of having a six pack. The main culprit? Cortisol. Cortisol is your stress hormone. Whenever your body goes through stress (mental or physical), your body secretes cortisol. In a normal situation, cortisol production only lasts for a short time, and afterward, all metabolic functions return to normal.

When your body experiences constant stress, it continuously secretes cortisol, and that's when cortisol becomes counterproductive to your body. Depending on how much cortisol you have, it can seriously affect your metabolic process and health, causing you to gain stubborn belly fat.

The six pack prescription? Sleep more, sleep deep, and sleep longer. 7-9 hours is ideal, but six is the minimum. Start by cutting out technology at least one hour before bed, keeping a regular sleep schedule, getting some sun early in the morning, and making sure you're actually spending 8-9 hours in bed.

The bottom line is your sleep hygiene is like your diet; it's either working for you or against you, multiplying or dividing your results.

LAW #56
BLOCK BLUE LIGHT

MOST OF US are on our phones or watching tv up until the second we decide it's time to go to sleep. The problem with this is that these devices emit blue light, which increases cortisol. Why is this important? Because when you increase cortisol, you decrease melatonin. So, not only will you have a harder time falling asleep, but your sleep quality will also decrease.

The best way to avoid subjecting yourself to blue light is to wear blue light blocking glasses. You can find a cheap pair on Amazon for $10-$20.

I try to get off my phone about two hours before bed. Reading a book (and journaling as we talked about) is a great way to relax and prepare your body for sleep. If you start doing this, you will notice a huge difference in how fast you are able to fall asleep, and your sleep quality will greatly increase.

LAW #57
TAKE COLD SHOWERS EVERY DAY

WHEN I FIRST heard about cold exposure for performance and recovery purposes in my days as an athlete, I brushed it off as a useless, new age fad.

It then resurfaced in my research for peak performance when I came across an article detailing the experience of sitting in a -264 degrees Fahrenheit cryotherapy machine for three minutes.

Undergoing this seemingly futuristic treatment is said to help your body incinerate calories, jolt your immune system back to life, and trigger a flood of mood-boosting endorphins, similar to a runner's high.

I want something that I can do at home and alas, I'm not yet a millionaire who can afford to buy a cryotherapy machine for myself, so I decided to look into more plebeian means to reap the same potential health benefits. That's how I came to discover the life-changing miracle of a cold shower.

The benefits of cold water therapy are numerous and fully backed by one metric fucktonne of research. This weird hack has been studied for generations, and even dates back as far as the time when the Spartans used it to recover after battle.

Today, professional athletes from all over use ice baths and cryotherapy to reduce inflammation and speed up recovery. Simply put, the cold exposure cleans you out by removing waste products like lactic acid that builds up from exercise.

Furthermore, when combined with alternating warm and cold water, these seemingly ridiculous showers clean out the lymphatic system. The lymphatic system helps carry waste out from your cells and is a major key in defending your body from unwanted infections. When it's blocked, you can get frequent colds and unexpected joint pain. These contrast showers — exposing your body to the cold water immediately after a warm shower — cleans out your lymph vessels and drastically improves your immune system.

Cold showers also help activate brown adipose tissue (BAT), which in turn generates heat, raises your metabolism, and burns off fat. It also seems to increase the amount of BAT in the body, leading to more calories burned and a leaner body.

Now as useful and sought-after as fat loss is, I was also intrigued by the potential productivity and performance enhancements that cold showers can deliver.

After extensive research I came to this conclusion: I definitely feel energized after a shower, but it wasn't the miracle cure for procrastination that many of my loyal cold shower enthusiasts have sworn by.

The biggest benefit that I've found is simply that a cold shower takes a lot of mental strength to accomplish. Point blank, they're hard. Like really, really hard.

And as research shows, people who do hard things early in the day tend to accomplish more and procrastinate less. To a cold shower virgin, the amount of willpower it takes to submerge oneself underneath a frozen waterfall may seem like that of a Shaolin Monk. Doing something that you are resistant to every day, immediately upon waking, takes an absurd amount of mental strength and discipline. It's the best way to start your day, and over time, these habits become automated and bleed into every area of your life.

The world is full of scary things; we're at our best when we tackle them bravely and with confidence, not when we've built up habits of shying away from things.

Think of it, quite literally, as stepping out of your comfort zone. So, set your alarm for five minutes earlier, and before you rush out of your shower, turn it all the way cold. It might be scary, but in no time, you'll have built it up as a habit.

LAW #58
GO DARK

WE SLEEP BETTER in the dark. Darkness helps to increase melatonin, which is considered the "sleep" hormone.

Our bodies produce the most amount of melatonin between the hours of 11 pm-3 am. This is why it's critical that you avoid all light during this time. Turn off the tv, turn off the night light and get off your phone. Just like your eyes, your skin has receptors that can pick up light. Therefore, if there is any hint of light in your bedroom, your skin could be picking it up, and this could be disrupting your sleep.

Try to buy "black-out curtains" to minimize any amount of light that might come through your window. If you have light coming through the bottom of your bedroom door, then roll up a towel or shirt to block it. Doing these things might seem insignificant, but it will make a big difference in your ability to fall asleep and stay asleep.

LAW #59
TURN UP THE HEAT

WHEN I WAS a kid, my mom would give me a nice warm bath every night before bed, and I would sleep like a baby, literally. You probably experienced the same thing. Why did this work?

When you take a hot bath or shower, the warm water lowers your body's core temperature. A drop in temperature helps signal to the body that it's time for bed.

The basic idea of taking a warm shower/bath at night is based on your core body temperature falling.

When your core body temperature falls, this signals the pineal gland to increase the production of melatonin. For most people, this happens between 10 pm and 11 pm.

If I plan on going to bed at 11 pm, then I will usually shower around 10 pm. This gives my body enough time to lower its core temperature once I am out of the shower, and by the time 11 pm comes, my body is ready to sleep.

PART 5

SUPPLEMENT LAWS

"My supplements are similar to my training - I always commit to being a better version of myself"

—Ronnie Coleman

SUPPLEMENTS HAVE GOTTEN a bad rap. There's tons of marketers and bodybuilders pushing low quality, underdosed supplements that essentially turn into very expensive pee.

There are also supplements which are backed by tonnes of research, proving to help speed up your six pack results. Here are our top choices.

LAW #60
TAKE MAGNESIUM

80% OF PEOPLE in the United States are deficient in magnesium. Magnesium is responsible for over 300 enzyme reactions in the body and is found in all of your tissue (i.e., bones, muscles, brain, etc.). Even though magnesium is an extremely impactful anti-stress mineral, it's quickly depleted from the body. This is likely the reason for magnesium deficiency being one of the most common mineral deficiencies in the world.

I had never supplemented with magnesium before, until one night, my roommate told me about his bedtime supplement routine. He would take magnesium 30 minutes before bed each night. I hadn't been sleeping well, so I tried taking magnesium one night to see if it helped. The biggest problem I have when I go to bed is turning my brain off. Taking magnesium before bed relaxed me and allowed my brain to calm down. Just this effect alone was extremely helpful.

Now, magnesium is not just helpful for sleep, but it helps with controlling stress and anxiety. Magnesium plays an important role in regulating GABA. Low levels of GABA (a neurotransmitter) have been connected to chronic pain, depression, and epilepsy. GABA imbalance has also been connected to panic disorder and sleep disturbances. The recommended amount of magnesium to take is

400-420 mg per day. I typically take magnesium 30 minutes before bed, as it helps to relax and de-stress my body and brain.

See our top magnesium product recommendations at petertzemis.com/magnesium

LAW #61
FISH OIL AND CURCUMIN

FIRMLY BELIEVE THAT everybody (not just those on the quest to six pack abs) should supplement with high-quality fish oil, as well as curcumin. These provide more health-boosting (and six pack carving) benefits than any other product you can buy. First off, both fish oil and curcumin have been shown to increase insulin sensitivity. If you have poor insulin sensitivity, you need to produce more of it when you eat a meal to "get the job done." This makes losing fat far more difficult. If insulin is high, your body is in storage mode, and energy mobilization isn't adequate. This means that the longer insulin stays up, the harder it is to drop fat.

By taking fish oil and curcumin daily, you help your body naturally defend against insulin resistance, making your six pack results 10x easier. Another big benefit of this duo is its ability to lower the acid load on the body. A highly acidic body has a negative impact on the hormonal profile (GH resistance, a decrease in IGF-1, issues with the insulin system, growth in cortisol, testosterone decrease, etc.), making it difficult to progress and reach low levels of body fat.

Lastly, evidence shows that curcumin can directly reduce abdominal fat storage by increasing leptin sensitivity and reducing cortisol release, specifically in the stomach area. In my experience, 6g of curcumin per day split into two or three doses is perfect for fighting off inflammation. I also consume two servings of fish oil per day in split doses (6-9g per dose).

See our top fish oil recommendations at
petertzemis.com/fishoil

LAW #62
SUPER DOSE ON VITAMIN D

I **N 1927, THERE** was an athletic controversy. The German Swimmers' Association had decided to use a sunlamp to boost their athletes' performance. Some believed this constituted "athletic unfairness."

You might be wondering how sitting under a sunlamp could be seen as doping? It's because it causes a steroid to be activated in the body. Vitamin D's metabolic product (calcitriol) is a secosteroid hormone, which is very similar to a steroid.

In fact, many classify vitamin D as a steroid hormone. Modern studies have shown that it can indeed be a performance-enhancing substance, especially if one is deficient. The fat-burning benefits of vitamin D are even better.

Research shows that adding vitamin D to a calorie-restricted diet may lead to better, faster weight loss. Low vitamin D levels are also associated with higher body fat in general. This leads to a vicious cycle of an increased inflammation response, which, in turn, helps add more belly fat.

How much should you take? Start with 2000-4000 IU per day and go from there. If you live in a colder climate where the sun disappears for 4-6 months during the winter, then you should be taking between 6000-8000 IU per day.

See our top vitamin D recommendations at
petertzemis.com/vitamind

LAW #63

NATURE'S FAT BURNER

UNFORTUNATELY, MANY FITNESS marketers and influencers take advantage of uninformed clients and followers and sell them garbage disguised as gold. I'm here to set the record straight. Fat burners are BS.

Ideally, if you were to take a "Fat Burning" supplement, you would want it to do three things:

1. Increase your basal metabolic rate. Your metabolic rate is how much energy your body burns throughout the day. Faster metabolism = faster fat loss.

2. Suppress your appetite. If you're constantly in a state of hunger, it's only a matter of time before you give in to your hunger and eat everything in sight. IF you can manage your hunger, you can sustain your nutrition plan long term. The biggest reason most diets fail is because people aren't able to stick to them long enough. If you can't stick to something long enough, then you will never reach your desired goal.

3. Give you more energy. If you could take a fat-burning supplement that gave you more energy, you would be more likely to exercise and move your body. More energy means moving your body more, which will burn more calories.

So is there a supplement that can do all of these things?

Yes. It's called caffeine.

Caffeine does a number of things that directly impacts fat loss. For one, caffeine stimulates lipolysis. Lipolysis causes the release of fatty acids into the bloodstream. Fat can't be burned unless it is actually released from the fat cell, and that is exactly what caffeine does.

Once the fatty acids are released into the bloodstream, they can be burned as energy.

There is a reason that most of the world drinks coffee in the morning: It wakes you up and gives you an energy kick. Like I said before, if you have more energy, then you will be much more likely to go workout and exercise.

One of the biggest benefits of caffeine, in my opinion, is the appetite suppressant effect it has. If you aren't hungry, you will be a lot less likely to snack or overeat. Caffeine is a natural appetite suppressant. If you are doing intermittent fasting, caffeine is your unfair advantage for longer fasts. When I'm fasting, I typically have 2-3 cups of coffee, and that will hold me over well into the afternoon.

So, if you aren't a coffee drinker or tea drinker, give it a try. You can always try caffeine pills if you don't like coffee or tea.

SUPPLEMENT WITH FIBER

FIBER ISN'T CONSIDERED "sexy," but it might actually be the number one six pack supplement since it does so much and is so inexpensive. A decades-long study published showed that consuming adequate quantities of dietary fiber can lead to improvements in gastrointestinal health, and a reduction in susceptibility to heart disease, and diabetes. Eating more fiber has also been associated with increased satiety and weight loss; which makes getting six pack abs a whole lot better.

There are two forms of dietary fiber: soluble and insoluble. Soluble fiber forms a gel-like substance that, among its many jobs, binds cholesterol and balances your blood sugar.

Insoluble fiber, on the other hand, absorbs water and keeps things moving along. The average American gets a sad 5–14 grams of fiber a day. Our lean, athletic Paleo ancestors put us to shame by getting a whopping 60 grams or more.

Use a fiber supplement to 'supplement' the deficiency. You can pick up a bulk-psyllium husk at your local grocery store (I prefer sugar-free orange Metamucil). Drink 1 serving 1-2x per day.

See our top fiber supplement recommendations at
petertzemis.com/fiber

NATURE'S NATURAL STEROID

I **F I TOLD** you there was an all-natural supplement you could take that would increase your muscle size, make you stronger, increase your performance and help you recover faster, would you take it? Of course, you would. This is exactly what creatine does.

Most people have heard of creatine, but most people don't understand exactly how it affects performance, recovery, strength, and muscle growth.

Creatine is one of the most researched supplements on the market. It is also one of the safest and most effective ones. Creatine is a naturally occurring substance that can be found in protein-rich foods like fish and meat. If your goal is to add muscle mass to your frame, then creatine is one of the most effective natural supplements you can take.

Let's take a look at some actual studies of the effects of creatine:

1. In one 6-week training study, the group who used creatine gained 4.4 pounds (2 kg) more muscle mass, on average, than the control group. https://www.ncbi.nlm.nih.gov/pubmed/10408330

2. Another comprehensive study found that when com-
   paring two controlled groups, there was a clear increase
   in lean muscle mass and overall strength with the group
   who was taking creatine. https://www.ncbi.nlm.nih.gov/
   pubmed/12433852

Here are some more benefits of creatine:

- Increased strength
- Increased muscle endurance
- Faster recovery
- Increased brain performance
- Less fatigue
- Helps control blood sugar

The most effective dose is 5-10 grams per day. You can buy creatine in powder or pill form. It's one of the cheapest supplements on the market, but it is the most effective.

See our top creatine recommendations at
petertzemis.com/creatine

LAW #66
MANAGE YOUR GUT HEALTH

HAVE YOU EVER gone on a night out and eaten a bunch of fried, fatty, or sugary foods? The next morning, you wake up feeling like garbage. You are slow, sluggish, and have brain fog. Maybe you are even more moody than usual. This happened to me every time I went out for my weekly "cheat meal."

Your gut is often called your "second brain." Your gut contains 500 million neurons. These neurons are connected to your brain through your nervous system.

Neurotransmitters that are produced in your brain control feelings and emotions. There is a specific neurotransmitter called serotonin. Serotonin contributes to feelings of happiness. A large proportion of serotonin is produced in your gut. So, if you think that what you eat doesn't affect your mood or happiness, you may want to think again.

The term "gut microbiome" refers to the microorganisms living in your intestines. A person has between 300 to 500 different species of bacteria living in their digestive tract. While some of these microorganisms can be harmful to our health, many of them are beneficial and vital for the body to function optimally and properly.

Having an unhealthy gut can lead to a number of issues. I

struggled with poor gut health for years, and I had no idea why. I would experience the following symptoms on almost a daily basis:

- Diarrhea
- Bloating after eating
- Gas
- Intense cravings for sugar
- Breakouts
- Weird skin irritations/rashes

Now, when I look back on this time in my life, there are a few reasons why I was experiencing these issues. I was eating and drinking a lot of foods with processed and artificial sweeteners. Just because something is classified as "low calorie" or "no-calorie," doesn't mean that it doesn't still have an impact on your body and your gut. I was drinking 1-2 diet cokes per day; I was taking pre-workouts that are loaded with artificial sweeteners and fillers. I was drinking sugar-free energy drinks. I was putting Splenda and calorie-free sweeteners in my coffee every morning.

All of these artificial sweeteners were wreaking havoc on my digestive system and killing all of the good bacteria in my gut. When you kill the good bacteria in your gut, you impair the body's ability to absorb nutrients, so even if you are eating healthy, your body will have a hard time absorbing nutrients and vitamins from the food.

The best way to ensure you avoid these issues is to try to reduce the consumption of processed foods and foods and drinks with artificial sweeteners. If you look at the ingredients on the nutrition labels of most of these sugar-free and diet drinks, they are loaded with fake chemicals. These chemicals destroy your gut bacteria and lead to a number of digestive issues in the long run.

Your gut also produces a neurotransmitter called gamma-aminobutyric acid (GABA), which helps to control feelings of fear and anxiety. An important thing you can do to ensure you have a healthy gut is to supplement with a probiotic. Studies in laboratory mice have shown that probiotics can help increase the production of GABA, which greatly helps to reduce anxiety and depression.

Probiotics are live bacteria that can help benefit gut health when eaten. To be an effective probiotic, it must contain live and active bacterial cultures. Always pick a probiotic with at least one billion colony-forming units and make sure it contains the genus Lactobacillus Bifidobacterium or Saccharomyces Boulardii. Don't stress, I know these are big words, but you can find all of this information out by looking at the back of the supplement label.

Another way to get more probiotics is by consuming more fermented foods. The following fermented foods are high in probiotics:

- Yogurts (with live and active cultures)
- Kombucha
- Sauerkraut
- Kimchi
- Kefir
- Miso
- Tempeh
- Certain cheeses - Gouda, mozzarella, cheddar and cottage cheese
- Pickles

If you can eat these foods daily, then you shouldn't worry about taking a probiotic supplement.

CONTROL CRAVINGS WITH GLUTAMINE

THE REASON WHY most people have sugar cravings is because of a change in blood sugar. If your blood sugar drops too low, you will have strong cravings for sweet and sugary foods. Therefore, if you can control blood sugar, you can control your cravings.

L-Glutamine is an amino acid that has been proven to help regulate blood sugar.

Another huge benefit of L-Glutamine is that it helps to increase the secretion of Human Growth Hormone (HGH). More HGH means more fat burning and a higher metabolic rate. You can increase your HGH levels by up to 300% by taking Glutamine every day. I advise taking 500mg of Glutamine three times per day with meals.

If you're having really strong sugar cravings, then you can take more servings until your cravings subside.

See our top glutamine recommendations at
petertzemis.com/glutamine

LAW #68
DRINK SODIUM BICARBONATE

WE ALL STRUGGLE with cravings from time to time. Whenever you have a craving for something, this is usually your body telling you that you're low or deficient in something, whether it be vitamins or minerals. More often than not, you're experiencing sugar cravings because your body is low on healthy salts.

Did you know that about 1% of our blood is salt? Salt gets a bad rap. We think of sodium as being bad for our health, but this couldn't be further from the truth. Your body needs sodium. Healthy salts are made of magnesium, potassium, calcium and sodium bicarbonates. These healthy salts are needed by the body for it to function optimally. Salt is also needed for proper electrolyte balance.

Now, like all things, anything in excess is bad. When it comes to salt, don't be afraid to salt your food.

Here is a trick I use to really kick sugar cravings:

Every time I feel a sugar craving coming on, I mix ½ tsp of sodium bicarbonate with eight ounces of water and gulp it down. Within seconds, my sugar cravings completely go away.

PART 6
SUCCESS LAWS

"Accountability is the glue that ties commitment to the result"
—BOB PROCTOR

BY THIS POINT in the book, you already have everything you need to get in the best shape of your life. If you take action and follow the nutrition and training laws, you will get results. Period. I could have saved myself a lot of time by skipping this part of the book, but I would have been doing you a big disservice because I know one thing…the best plan in the world means nothing if it isn't followed.

As a professional fitness coach, I've realized I can give someone the best information in the world, but if it isn't followed and no action is taken, then it means nothing. This is where accountability comes in.

There are no guarantees in life, but you can make damn sure that you put as many safeguards in place as you can to keep you accountable and hold your feet to the fire.

I have a fitness coach. Yes, I am a fitness coach writing a book on fitness and I have a fitness coach. Why? Accountability. I love food just as much as everyone else. Some days, I would rather drive to an all-you-can-eat sushi buffet instead of going to the gym…but I don't, and this is where accountability comes in.

Accountability creates responsibility. At the end of the day, you are responsible for your actions and the result of those actions. Every Saturday morning, I send my coach my current photos and weight. If I am heavier or look fatter than the week before, I am going to have to explain what happened and why it happened. This accountability I have to my coach makes it a lot harder for me to cheat on my diet or skip the gym.

Now, you don't need to hire a coach. However, having accountability will greatly assist you with keeping you on the path to success. I suggest finding an accountability partner. This can be your spouse, a friend, a co-worker, brother, sister, etc. The beautiful thing is that they don't have to know anything about fitness. It can be something as simple as telling your wife that by this time next week, you are going to weigh 200lbs (assuming your weight was 203lbs). And if you don't hit your goal, you pay her $50 or take her to a fancy restaurant. You get the point.

This process can be as fun as you want to make it. Just realize, having accountability is the fastest way to guarantee you reach your goal. After a few weeks of training and eating in a calorie deficit, it can be really easy to convince yourself to pull over into that Krispy Kreme parking lot and order a dozen donuts. After all, we are only human. But, if you know there will be consequences for your actions than the likelihood of this happening will be a lot less likely.

LAW #69

KNOW YOUR HORMONES

CHRISTMAS EVE 2019, I decided to get my bloodwork done. I was recommended to a hormone replacement clinic by a friend who had been dealing with some issues associated with having low testosterone. He told me to go get checked just to see if there were any issues. I was 30 years old, so I thought it was a waste of time, but I went anyway because I was curious to see where my levels were.

Four days later, I got a call from the office to go over my results. All of my bloodwork markers came back good...except for one thing. My testosterone. My testosterone had come back at 242 ng/dL. What does that mean? Essentially, I was chemically castrated and I had no idea.

Testosterone levels typically range from 300ng/DL - 1200ng/DL. 300 is extremely low, and 1200 is considered on the high end of optimal.

In case this might be an issue for you, here are some signs that you may have low testosterone:

- Low sex drive
- Difficulty getting an erection
- Low semen count

- Feeling tired and fatigued
- Hair loss
- Increased body fat
- Loss of muscle mass
- Decreased bone mass
- Depression
- Mood swings
- Smaller testicles
- Poor sleep
- Little or no energy

When you think of someone having low T, you will likely think of an older guy who is way past his prime. You never think of a young, healthy guy having low T. At 30 years old, I was supposed to be in my prime, but my hormone levels said otherwise.

Up until this point in my life, I had felt pretty good. My energy levels were normal; my sleep was decent, my sex drive was normal (or so I thought), I would get moody from time to time but thought it was normal. There were really no obvious red flags.

When I finally sat down with the doctor to talk about possible options moving forward, he said something that made a lot of sense. He said, "you've been feeling normal, but it's because you don't know what it's like to feel optimal." After a second, I thought to myself…maybe he's right. Maybe I had become so used to feeling what I thought was normal that I had no idea what it was like to feel optimal.

I don't know about you, but I want to live an optimal life, not a normal one. Unfortunately, many men go through life with low testosterone and never realize it because they think it's "normal." That was me until I got tested.

I started testosterone replacement therapy (TRT) the following week. I didn't feel a difference for the first 30 days. Once I started month two of treatment, I started to feel a huge difference. The first thing I noticed was that I was sleeping better. Sleep is critical for getting lean and building muscle. I also noticed I was waking up with "morning wood." My energy levels were high and I actually wanted to go to the gym whereas before I would force myself to go. Before I started treatment, I would have normal workouts, but never great workouts. Again, I thought that was normal. But now, every time I go to the gym, my muscles swell within minutes of training. Every workout feels amazing. I also noticed I was able to drop body fat faster. Before I would need to diet extremely hard and go very low with my calories to make progress whereas now I drop fat almost effortlessly. Don't get me wrong, you still need to eat right and train hard to lose fat, but it's much easier when your body is working optimally.

After 6 weeks of being on TRT, my testosterone levels went from 242ng/dL to 902ng/dL.

I think the biggest difference since being on treatment is the change in my mood and overall outlook on life. I have never suffered from depression. In the past, I had good days and bad days just like anyone else, but for the most part, I always thought positive and had hope. I still have my share of good days and bad days, but my outlook is so much better. I wake up happy and excited for the day ahead. My ambition is through the roof!

The truth is, I probably would've never written this book if I hadn't started TRT, because my drive and ambition were so low. Before, I literally felt like I needed to watch three hours worth of motivation videos before doing anything, and now the motivation and drive are just automatic.

Now, don't get me wrong, testosterone replacement therapy isn't a miracle. You can't continue to just eat whatever you want and not train and expect to feel amazing. Everything works together. If you have healthy testosterone levels, then you will feel good. When you feel good, you want to exercise and workout. When you workout, you want to make healthy food choices.

It's important to note, testosterone replacement therapy (TRT) is not the same as taking steroids. There are a lot of idiots that will say it's the same thing, but they are uninformed and uneducated. Even though testosterone is considered an anabolic steroid, when used in a therapy dosage, it's completely safe. Testosterone causes problems when you take too much. Pro bodybuilders often abuse it and take super-physiological doses, and that's why they can experience problems. The objective with TRT is to bring your testosterone levels to an optimal level for you.

If you happened to have a vineyard, you could have the perfect weather conditions and the best "supplements," but if the soil is rotten, you won't grow a whole lot. The same is true with your body: You can have the best coach, perfect training, and a fantastic nutrition regimen, the best supplements, but if your body is "rotten," you will make very little progress, if any.

"Rotten" means "not optimally healthy," and I'm referring to your hormones. If you push your body to work in non-optimal conditions, be ready to experience some pushback. That's why the first thing I have my private coaching clients do as soon as we start working together is to get their blood work done to see where their hormone levels are at.

Here's what I recommend you get tested (regardless of your age) once a year:

- Comprehensive Metabolic Panel
- CBC
- Lipid Panel

- FREE Testosterone and Total Testosterone
- Estradiol Sensitive
- DHEA-S
- TSH
- Free T3
- Reverse T3
- PSA
- LH
- FSH

LAW #70
MAKE A NOT-TO DO LIST

YOU WERE CREATED to live an amazing life. Don't ever question that. You need to believe it deep down inside yourself. Living an elite life is a choice the same way living a normal life is a choice. Only you can decide which you want.

You can start making better choices and decisions immediately, regardless of where you are in your life. I'm a positive person and don't like to use scare tactics or fear to motivate people, but I want to bring this to your attention. You're not where you are in your life by accident. Your current situation is the result of the choices you have made up until this point.

> *"I am not a product of my circumstances. I am a product of my decisions."*
>
> ~ STEPHEN COVEY

In life, it's important to make the right choices, but equally important to avoid making the wrong ones.

This is why I give myself a set of rules to live by and this is why I created the NOT To-Do List. This is a list of all of the actions you absolutely should not do to avoid setbacks and reach your goal.

Here's my Six Pack Abs NOT To-Do List:

1. I will not eat outside of my daily caloric intake
2. I will get my 10,000 steps every day
3. I will not sit for more than 4 hours per day
4. I will not skip the gym
5. I will not hit the snooze button
6. I will not eat before 12 pm or after 8 pm
7. I will not keep sweet and tempting foods in my house
8. I will not drink alcohol Mon-Fri

The thought of creating an "anti-rules" list may seem odd, but you'll come to see how avoiding certain actions will allow you to make progress and you will achieve your goals faster than you ever thought possible.

Before continuing on to the next law, create your own NOT To-Do List.

LAW #71

WEIGH YOURSELF DAILY

I STARTED WEIGHING MYSELF every day when I lived in Toronto. I had just moved there, and I told my roommate and friend that I wanted to drop 20lbs. He wanted to drop a few pounds himself, so we decided to keep each other accountable. We kept a digital scale in the living room, and every morning, we would weigh ourselves and write our weight down on a whiteboard. This was our way of keeping each other accountable, and guess what? It worked.

Ever since then, I weigh myself first thing every single morning after I go to the bathroom and before I have anything to eat or drink. This is something that effortlessly helps to keep me on track.

I have my private clients do the same thing. Why? Because it puts your goal (six pack abs) to the front of your mind as soon as you wake up. This ensures that every decision you make during the day and night will be somewhat influenced by the fact that you will have to step on the scale the next morning. Nobody likes seeing their weight go up, so you will be much less likely to overeat and go overboard with your calories. It almost becomes like a game. You always want to beat the previous day and see your weight drop a little lower every morning.

Now, your weight fluctuates every day. Weight fluctuations are based on many factors (water, salt, food volume, etc.) As long as the trend continues downward each week, you know you're moving in the right direction.

The best way to track your weight is to take a weekly average. You do this by adding all seven days of your weight together and dividing by seven.

For example:

Monday: 207 lbs

Tuesday: 207.8 lbs

Wednesday: 206.9 lbs

Thursday: 206.4 lbs

Friday: 207 lbs

Saturday: 206 lbs

Sunday: 205.8 lbs

207 + 207.8 + 206.9 + 206.4 + 207 + 206 + 205.8 = 206.7

So your weekly average is 206.7 lbs. The following week, compare your new weekly average to the previous week's average. The trend should be going down if you are making progress. If not, then you need to take a closer look at your calorie intake.

LAW #72
SEEK OUT ACCOUNTABILITY

THIS LAW WILL be the most important law you read. It has the power to change your life if you apply it.

When I was 17 years old, I hired my first coach. I was obsessed with bodybuilding and I wanted to compete in my first bodybuilding show. My coach trained me in the gym, helped me with my nutrition, and showed me how to pose. He had the knowledge, the experience, and most importantly, he had a long list of successful athletes and bodybuilders he'd worked with. The reason I trusted him was because his results spoke for themselves. I ended up getting 2nd place in the teen division and 4th place in the men's division. It was an amazing experience that I'll never forget.

Early on in my life, I realized that having a coach was my unfair advantage. Instead of making mistakes that cost time and money, I could find someone who had done it all, seen it all, and who had helped others reach their goals. I could hire them as my personal coach and fast forward my results.

The best athletes in the world have an entire team of coaches they work with. Mental coaches, strength coaches, nutrition coaches, etc. The reason they're the best in the world is because they realize they don't know everything, and to optimize performance, they need to work with experts in their field.

Have you heard of a guy named "The Rock?" Maybe you've seen a few of his movies. Did you know he has a coach who creates his weight-training program and another coach who helps him with his nutrition? It's the reason why he looks the way he does on the big screen.

I have multiple coaches. One of the reasons you are reading this book is because I hired a writing coach to help me. I have a business coach, an MMA coach, and I have my fitness coach who helps keep me on track with my diet and training.

Now, this might sound unusual to some of you. Why would someone who is an expert on fitness hire someone else to train him?

ACCOUNTABILITY.

When you know someone you respect is counting on you, you show up and do the work. This translates into training, business, dating, therapy, or nearly anything else. Hiring a coach makes it nearly impossible to fail.

The mere thought of having to be responsible for our actions, which will then be evaluated, makes us want to crush it day in and day out. In addition, the wisdom of an experienced coach allows us to overcome many pitfalls that would've happened if we had gone at it alone.

Do you honestly believe that Luke would've defeated Darth Vader and Darth Sidious without Yoda? If there's an area of your life you want to level up in, you can go at it alone and take the long way, or you can take the shortcut to success and hire a coach. It'll be one of the best investments you'll ever make.

Now, you might be thinking, this sounds great and all Stephen, but I can't afford a coach. Let me try to change your perspective.

I'll give you an example. What if you were a salesman for a

pharmaceutical company. But you're 40 pounds overweight. Your clothes fit tight, and this makes you self-conscious about how you look. Because you are self conscious, you're not as confident when you try to sell. This directly impacts your ability to close sales, and it hurts your income. Now, you are smart, so you buy and read this book, and you remember law #72 - Seek out Accountability. So you hire a fitness coach and drop the 40 pounds in 12 weeks and build some muscle. You feel better than ever and it shows in how you walk, talk, and sell. Because you have confidence in yourself, you end up closing more deals and making more money. Hiring a coach ends up being the best investment you've ever made. Not only do you look and feel better, but you are making more money.

Let's look at another scenario. Maybe you're a 25-year-old guy who has been single a while. You're 20 pounds overweight and a little chubby. The reason you're single is because you lack the confidence to go talk to that pretty girl you always see at Starbucks. This girl, let's call her "Jessica," could potentially be your future wife, but you'll never know because you never talk to her. You're insecure about how you look and you miss opportunities to talk to girls. Now, you're smart and remember reading about this law in the book, so you hire a fitness coach. You get lean and now have a six pack. You look good, feel good, and are confident. You see Jessica at Starbucks again and decide to say hello. Fast forward one year later, and you are proposing to her on a beach in Hawaii. That would have never happened if you didn't decide to take action and get in shape. This one decision changes the entire direction and course of your life.

So, in the end, you can't afford NOT to hire a coach. Change your thinking, change your perspective, and you will change your life.

TAKE WEEKLY MEASUREMENTS AND PHOTOS

SUCCESS LEAVES CLUES. Having worked with thousands of people over the years with varying goals, I've noticed a trend: The clients who lost the most weight and had the biggest physical transformation tracked everything. They tracked their calories, they tracked their weight, they took weekly photos and measurements. They were meticulous about tracking. This allowed them to not only see their changes (which fuelled their motivation), but it allowed them to course-correct quickly and make adjustments if something was off.

This is why all of my clients are required to track everything. When we do our weekly check-ins, I look at their weight and how it has changed from the previous week. I look at their photos to see if there are any differences to the week prior. Depending on how much their body changed or didn't change, I adjust their calorie and macronutrient intake. We track everything.

"What gets measured, gets managed." We can't make adjustments if we don't know what to adjust. Now, even though I advocate weighing yourself every day, the scale is not the only metric we use. If you only measure your progress by the number on the scale, then you are setting yourself up for failure. Your weight can also fluctuate 5-10lbs on a given day. According to the scale, it looks like you gained weight, but maybe you are just holding water because you had more sodium or carbs yesterday. Or maybe you haven't gone to the bathroom yet. Many things can affect your weight.

Here are the best methods you can use to track your progress and ensure you are on the right path:

Take pictures - Either have someone take them of you or stand in front of a mirror. You can do it in your boxers, underwear, or a bathing suit. Take a front shot, side shot and back shot. Print them out and put them in an album or keep them in your phone so you can compare photos from week to week. Every week take new photos, this way, you'll be able to make comparisons and see how your body is changing.

Take measurements - Grab a measuring tape and, in the morning, take the following measurements and write them down: Neck, chest, and waist (belly button). Make sure to take them at the same time every week and in the same location. Use a freckle or other skin marker to help locate the same area if possible.

The best indication that you're on the right track is if your clothes fit better. Whenever I am able to go down a notch on my belt, I know my waist is getting smaller, even if the scale hasn't moved. If my shirts are feeling a little looser, I know my body is changing.

LAW #74
HAVE A POST-SIX-PACK PLAN

WHENEVER I HAVE an initial consultation with someone before we start working together, I always say this: "this is not just a 12-week transformation. What good is it if I help you get in the best shape of your life, but when the 12 weeks are over, you go back to your old habits and you lose the results you have gotten?" Once you decide to get in better shape and start working towards getting six pack abs, the body will change very quickly. But, to maintain your new body, you need to make your new healthy habits a lifestyle.

On occasion, I get clients who have achieved their goal, only to lose it a few months later. They return to their former overweight selves, after a little bit of glory, wondering what the hell happened. Often, it's a product of a poor self-image and bad environment. Other times though, it's simply a product of poor planning.

One of the biggest mistakes 99.9% of people make once they have hit their goal of being at a certain body fat % is they stuff their faces with food. There is nothing wrong with enjoying yourself and overindulging on the foods you love, but you can't allow that to happen too often or you will end up right back where you started.

I remember when I competed in my teen bodybuilding show, all I could think about was stuffing my face after the show was over.

One night of binge eating turned into one week of binge eating and one week turned into multiple weeks of binging and within a few short weeks, I was literally right where I started. 16 weeks of intense dieting and training were destroyed. It was depressing, to say the least. You must avoid this at all costs.

It's critical that you have a plan once you reach your goal.

I recommend a reverse taper diet. As you get leaner, your metabolism down-regulates (slows down). If your metabolism is slower and you start overeating, your body will put on fat pretty quickly. To dodge this, you need to slowly increase your calories on a weekly basis, while simultaneously cutting back on excessive exercise. When you do this in a slow and controlled manner, your metabolism will start to increase.

When your metabolism increases, you can increase your calories a little bit more each week, and your body will actually use that newly reintroduced energy (calories) more effectively. The goal is maintaining a shapely physique while being able to eat a good amount of calories.

Here's your post-six-pack plan: Every week, add 100 calories back into your diet and cut your cardio or exercise by about 10%. Do this for 6-8 weeks, and you'll have restored your metabolism while keeping your six pack (by training your body to eat more food). If you see you're adding body fat and your weight increases, then pull back and lower your calories until your metabolism adjusts to the calories you are consuming. When you can maintain your weight for one week, then it's safe to start increasing calories.

DRESS BETTER

CALL ME A little princess, but I've always found that I'm more motivated to become (and stay) shredded when I dress better. Oftentimes the clothes show off my physique, so if I'm a fat slob, then I'm gonna look like crap, which motivates me even further.

More important though, putting on a well-thought-out look sets the tone for the day. I tell my subconscious mind that I'm ready to take on the day. Science backs this up as well. People who dress well tend to have better posture, be more productive, and yes, be in better shape.

As we know, people judge you very quickly. We often forget that we are also people and judge quickly too. When we see ourselves dressed as a fat slob, often our actions come to reflect that. When we dress well, the last thing we want to do is pig out and stuff our faces. Go put on a suit and then try and put down pints of ice cream, pizza and whatever crap you crave. It's impossible.

LAW #76

KNOW YOUR CRAVING TYPE

THE WORD CRAVING is used very superficially in the fitness industry. The majority of fitness professionals associate the word craving with food (pizza, pancakes, ice cream, etc.) Often, though we are craving something much deeper than that, and trying to cope by filling the void with unnecessary calories.

We end up being the walking dead, in a state of living where our deepest core desires have gone unfulfilled, forcing us to self-medicate with pseudo cravings. When we redefine and figure out our true craving, we play offense instead of defense. Next time you feel like bingeing out, take a second to examine what your body and mind are truly craving.

THE TEN TYPES OF CRAVINGS:

Safety - Now this doesn't include physical safety (as many first world readers will have that covered.) It includes status safety, job safety, and emotional safety. Identifying and acknowledging these legitimate threats are the first step to understanding where a large degree of stress comes from.

Mobility - Mobility is a key fundamental law of successful humans. If we can't move because we are sick, we get stressed and feel unfulfilled. But it's not only physical mobility - it can be economical as well. If you are working hard to move up, but haven't you can have some serious stress and look for coping mechanisms.

Movement - Healthy humans crave movement. When we sit at a desk all day, we rarely get the movement we need. Movement is closely linked to psychological health healing to manage/mitigate anxiety, depression, and stress.

Love & Relationships - As a pack-oriented animal we have a biological need for tight-knit relationships. Unfortunately, we have leaned towards isolation more than ever. When we feel isolated or unloved, we feel deprived and search for a method to cope, often turning to alcohol or food.

Social Acceptance - Being rejected by a social group is one of the worst psychological things that can happen to a human being. That's because, in all of our history, social acceptance has been synonymous with our survival. Having a social circle is one of the easiest ways to mitigate stress and enjoy life.

Purpose - When we struggle to make our mark and find our why, it can lead to significant stress. Often we search for escapes in the form of food to cope. Finding your purpose is one of the most liberating things you can do for your abs.

Health & vitality - Failing to properly take care of oneself leads to severe mental and physical stress. It also leads to the never-ending cycle of feeding yourself unnecessary food which makes you even more unhealthy.

Autonomy - Humans crave independence and freedom. When we feel like we are oppressed, stress levels rise, and we begin to crave independence again.

Pseudo Cravings - Often this is what people think about when they think of cravings. Often these foods though are not the answer. Instead, they are intact coping mechanisms trying to fill a void of the nine other desires on this list. It's important to note that these cravings are not bad - they are simply information.

Self-actualization - As humans, we crave innovation, challenge, and discovery. When things are stifled, we often crave for lack of self-actualization.

I'll mention it again: Unfulfilled core human cravings trigger superficial cravings. Rather than defending yourself from superficial cravings (processed food) you can engage in behaviors that create fulfillment in your core human cravings. Once those are filled (or at the very least, attempted to be filled) the original pseudo-cravings will be gone.

TAKE ACTION AND NEVER GIVE UP

I HATE TO REHASH generic personal-improvement principles, but here's the truth - nothing happens without action. You can lead a horse to water, but you can't make it drink. The same principles apply when it comes to transforming your body. All of the knowledge and information shared in this book means nothing if you don't apply it. You know the saying "knowledge is power"? Well, that's actually bullshit. Applied knowledge is power. You can have all the knowledge in the world if it isn't put into practice, it's worthless.

Reading is not considered taking action. It's not even considered learning. It's considered reading. Learning is a product of experience. Experience is a part of taking action. Use the laws and go take action now. If you want to be at the top (top 1-10%), you will have to do things differently than 90-99% of people.

Before I sign off, let me remind you of two things:

1. You need to really earn your rest days. There will be days that you will feel motivated, focused, well-rested, and have a full day without interruptions to work on your goal. Other days you'll have none of that. On those days, just do something and try to feel good about it. This is better than doing nothing and feeling bad about it. (or doing nothing and feeling okay about it). Just because you can't give it 100% on that specific day, doesn't mean your 50% time investment (or even 50% effort) won't pay some future dividends. Don't give yourself a "rest day" simply because you are lazy that day. Earn your rest days.

2. You will regret not trying far more than failing. Not trying, you will always wonder, what if?

These things will keep you up at night, the kind of stuff that makes for a midlife crisis, and the kind of stuff that you will regret for the rest of your life. When someone isn't sure if they should go "all in" on whatever their goal/dream is, this is what I ask them to consider - what the hell are they going to do instead, plan B?

Plan B is not only uninspiring, it isn't a plan at all. "Plan B" is simply not trying Plan A. Rather than wasting time pretending that you have a suitable "Plan B," I encourage you to pursue plan A and fall flat on your face. Learn from it and move forward. Be all in. Burn the boats.

Even if you fail miserably (you won't), you'll never regret it. I promise.

BONUS

THE ULTIMATE SIX PACK SUPPLEMENT STACK

PLEASE SEE THE note at the end of this chapter...

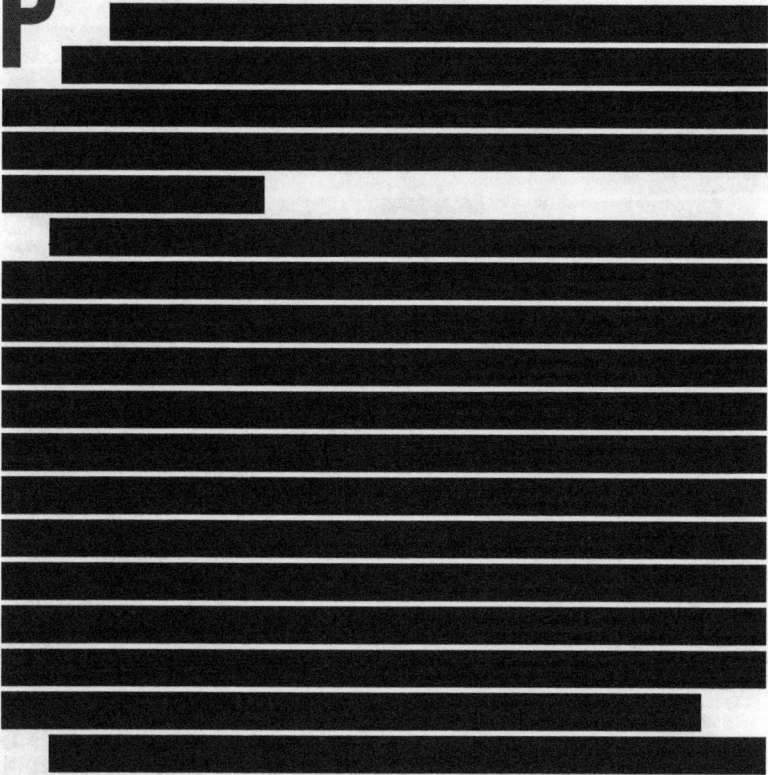

STEPHEN CAMPOLO & PETER TZEMIS

Unfortunately, this law was removed by our publishing lawyer because it was deemed too controversial.

However, based on our publishing lawyers recommendation, here's what we need you to do if you want access to this...

1. Go to this link: https://petertzemis.com/law78/
2. Sign up with your name and email.

Once that's complete, we'll send you the controversial, never-before-seen BANNED chapter from The 77 Laws of Six Pack Abs.

Also known as the 78th law.

To access it, you'll need the PDF password: BANNED.

Unfortunately, we can't keep this up forever, because we don't know how long until big brother finds out and forces us to take it down.

So I urge you to act fast, before it's too late.

ADDITIONAL READING:

Cold therapy:
https://romanfitnesssystems.com/articles/cold-therapy/

Boosting Testosterone:
https://romanfitnesssystems.com/
articles/testosterone-sex-drive/

Hormones for Fat Loss:
https://romanfitnesssystems.com/
articles/lose-stubborn-fat/

Magnesium:
https://romanfitnesssystems.com/articles/magnesium/

Creatine:
https://romanfitnessssystems.com/articles/creatine/

Gut health:
https://romanfitnesssystems.com/articles/poop/

Leg Training:
https://romanfitnessssystems.com/
articles/chicken-legs-training/

Intermittent Fasting:
https://romanfitnesssystems.com/
articles/intermittent-fasting-101/

How to Change Eating Habits:
https://romanfitnesssystems.com/articles/eating-habits/

ABOUT THE AUTHORS

Stephen is a former fat kid turned weight loss expert. He lost 100lbs naturally through sheer willpower and determination. In 2003 he started his journey, running every night along the streets of long island, NY. Within 3 months, he lost nearly 60lbs. But the result was far from the herculean look he dreamed of. Instead, he ended up with a bunch of excess skin and no muscle. So he picked up a FLEX magazine with Arnold on the cover and started to learn everything he could about building the ultimate male physique.. Hundreds of hours later and thousands of pounds of iron lifted, he had made it. Stephen has competed in natural bodybuilding shows and has worked with some of the top trainers and nutrition coaches in the country. Today he shares his knowledge with the world, and currently serves as the top trainer and advisor to various celebrities, CEO's and has created fitness programs for the U.S. military. For more about Stephen, head over to 77laws.com/stephen.

Peter Tzemis is a bestselling author and internet marketer. He started his journey in fitness in 2015, learning how to carve the body of a greek god. While getting his Bachelor of Health Sciences, he wrote his first fitness book, Anabolic Stretching, which sold over 5000 copies in the first few months. Since then he's gone on to write multiple books in the health space and become a partner in one of the internet's most prominent health and fitness websites: roman-fitnesssytems.com. Today, he actively plays a role in selling over $50,000,000 worth of online products in a variety of niches. He also blogs all his life lessons at petertzemis.com and marketing lessons at beatyourcontrol.com. For more about Peter, head over to 77laws.com/peter.

www.ingramcontent.com/pod-product-compliance
Lightning Source LLC
Chambersburg PA
CBHW030246030426
42336CB00009B/280